PROCEDURES IN PRACTICE

PROCEDURES IN PRACTICE

Articles published in
the *British Medical Journal*
Published by the British Medical Association
Tavistock Square, London WC1H 9JR

First Edition 1981
Second Impression 1983
Third Impression 1985

ISBN 0 7279 0075 7

Printed in England by The Devonshire Press, Barton Road, Torquay.
Typesetting by Bedford Typesetters Ltd, Bedford.

Preface

by the Editor
British Medical Journal

In the early years after graduation every clinician has to acquire the practical skills of his specialty. Few doctors have the ability to remember every step of a procedure after seeing a single demonstration. This series of articles (first published in the *BMJ* and now collected together with minor revisions to take account of comments by readers after the initial publication) is intended to provide a step-by-step guide for doctors making their first attempts at the common procedures in hospital practice. We hope that the information will make life easier both for doctors and for their long-suffering patients.

STEPHEN LOCK

1981

Contents

Contents

Contents

KIDNEY BIOPSY

RICHARD McGONIGLE   PAUL SHARPSTONE

Indications

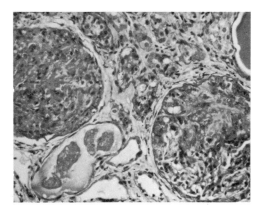

Patients with renal glomerular disease may present with similar clinical features yet have conditions ranging from the trivial to the life-threatening. Their prognosis and treatment depend on the renal pathology, and histological examination of the kidney is often the only way to make the diagnosis. Needle biopsy, however, provides a sample of only about 20 of the 2 000 000 glomeruli, so is unhelpful and may give misleading results in patchy conditions such as chronic pyelonephritis. It is most valuable in assessing and, in particular, indicating the prognosis of patients with diffuse glomerular disease. The table summarises the principal indications for its use.

Principal indications for kidney biopsy

Clinical syndrome	Indications for biopsy
Asymptomatic proteinuria	Protein excretion more than 1 g/24 h Red blood cells in urine Impaired renal function
Recurrent isolated haematuria	Intravenous urography and cystoscopy do not show source Proteinuria also present
Acute nephritic syndrome	Persisting oliguria
Nephrotic syndrome	Adults: unless cause is apparent from extrarenal manifestations Children: only if haematuria also present, or if proteinuria persists after trial of corticosteroid
Acute renal failure	No obvious precipitating cause Renal-tract obstruction excluded
Chronic renal failure	Radiographically normal kidneys

Contraindications

Contralateral kidney inadequate

Only one kidney

Haemorrhagic tendency

Platelet count $< 100 \times 10^9/l$

Prothrombin time $\geqslant 16$ s

Kidneys shrunken

Laceration of the kidney may cause haemorrhage, which may lead to nephrectomy. The risk is small but should always be kept in mind, and biopsy should be done only if the other kidney is adequate. A single kidney or major abnormality of the contralateral kidney are contraindications, as is any haemorrhagic tendency, including advanced uraemia. The platelet count should be over $100 \times 10^9/l$ (100 000/mm^3) and the prothrombin time less than 16 seconds. Biopsy should not be done on shrunken kidneys because they are difficult to locate, the histology is often non-specific, and, in any case, the result is unlikely to provide information of any therapeutic relevance.

Kidney biopsy

Technique

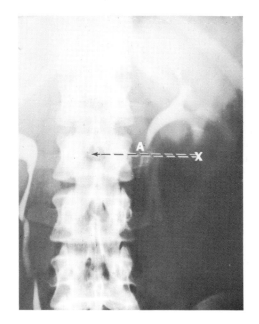

Premedication with intravenous diazepam makes the procedure less unpleasant for the patient; general anaesthesia is required only for infants and young children. A firm surface is needed, so have bed boards under the mattress. Place the patient prone with his head turned away (most patients do not want to watch), his arms abducted, and his forearms beside his head. Put a rolled-up towel (about 10 cm in diameter) under the patient's abdomen between the rib cage and pelvis.

The preferred site is the centre of the lower pole of the left kidney. This avoids the major renal vessels and is likely to contain more cortex than medulla. On an intravenous urogram film measure the distance (A) of this point from the lumbar spinous processes. The bony landmarks are the tips of the dorsal processes of the lumbar spine and lower border of the 12th rib. Palpate and mark these on the patient's skin. Then draw a line (B) vertically downwards from the 12th rib at distance A from the spine. Measuring the length of B on the x-ray film is unreliable because of radiological distortion, so simply choose a site along B 2 cm below the lower border of the 12th rib. If you fail to locate the kidney there, go higher still. Ultrasound examination gives more accurate localisation of the kidney but is unnecessary in most cases.

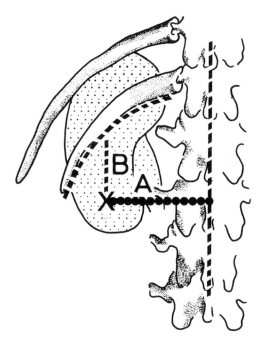

Wear sterile gloves and stand at the left side of the patient. Prepare the skin and locally anaesthetise the skin and subcutaneous tissues, then use a 17 cm, 1·1 mm (19 G) exploring needle to find the kidney. Insert it into the lumbar muscles and then advance it 5 mm at a time until a definite swing with respiration shows that the point is within the kidney. Ask the patient to hold his breath in inspiration each time you move the needle and to take a deep breath out and in after each advance. Do not restrict movement of the needle while the patient is breathing—handle it only while he is holding his breath. The kidney is about 5-8 cm deep; after locating it, inject local anaesthetic along the track while withdrawing the needle.

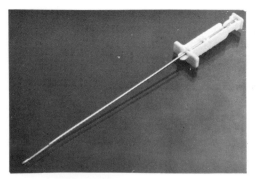

To take the biopsy specimen the Vim-Silverman needle, with the Franklin modification, and the Tru-Cut disposable needle (Travenol Laboratories Ltd) are equally effective. We shall describe the Tru-Cut technique. The 11·4 cm needle is suitable for most patients, but use the 15 cm one for larger patients.

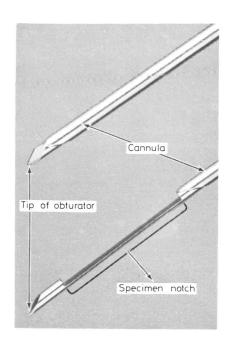

Make a nick in the skin with the point of a scalpel blade and then advance the biopsy needle, with the cannula closed over the obturator, stepwise as with the exploring needle. A large arc of swing usually shows that the kidney has been located, but beware the patient who uses his chest more than his diaphragm when asked to breathe deeply. When the swing is small it is easy to penetrate the full thickness of the kidney, and the specimen obtained will comprise only fat or blood clot. In these patients correct location of the point of the needle depends on feeling the resistance of the capsule and the "give" on penetrating it. The disposable needle is sharp and the change in resistance slight, so, for sensitive control, hold it low down by the shaft rather than by its handle. Another indication of reaching the kidney is the transmission of arterial pulsation. A small jerk with each respiratory movement means that the tip of the needle is just scraping the capsule and should be advanced a little further. If the needle moves only at the extreme of inspiration it is probably being struck by the lower pole and should be reinserted higher up.

When you are satisfied that the tip is *just* within the kidney ask the patient to hold his breath in inspiration. Then tap the obturator handle in, push the cannula smartly down the length of its travel to cut the specimen, keeping the obturator handle firmly fixed with the other hand, and finally withdraw the needle with the cannula closed over the obturator. The last three manoeuvres must be made while the patient is holding his breath, so practise them on a ripe pear first!

The specimen

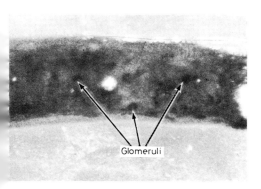

A successful biopsy produces a strip of kidney up to 20 mm long. Immunofluorescence microscopy is carried out on fresh tissue, while routine and electron microscopy require appropriate fixatives. When all these techniques are available the specimen must be divided into three, so examine each part with a hand lens or dissecting microscope and make sure that all contain glomeruli. If there is any doubt about their adequacy obtain another specimen rather than risk having to repeat the whole performance later when you receive a histology report reading "medulla only."

Aftercare and complications

Check pulse and blood pressure

Keep patient in bed

Beware haemorrhage

The patient should remain in bed for 24 hours and have his pulse and blood pressure checked hourly for four hours and then at four-hour intervals.

The most important complication is haemorrhage, which may be perirenal, causing loin pain and sometimes a palpable mass as well as the signs of blood loss; or intrapelvic, causing persisting heavy haematuria and sometimes clot retention. More minor haematuria is common and usually settles quickly. Continuing haemorrhage should be treated by blood transfusion and sedation. Exploration of the kidney is only rarely required.

LARYNGOSCOPY

M J AL-KHALED   PHILIP H BEALES

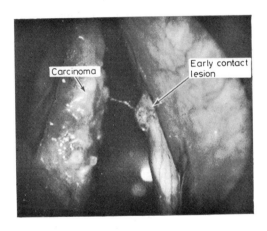

Laryngoscopy is the method of examining the larynx from above by direct vision. It should always be preceded by an inspection of the exterior of the larynx in the neck, and of the movements on deglutition, when the larynx normally moves upwards. The larynx moves downwards on inspiration in laryngeal stenosis and is immobile in tracheal stenosis. Palpation of the larynx in the neck will disclose any broadening and tenderness that may indicate perichondritis of the thyroid cartilage.

Indications

Indications

Persistent hoarseness

Stridor

Thyroidectomy

Dysphagia

Earache

Contraindications

Acute inflammation of the throat causing trismus

Acute epiglottitis

Diagnosis—The commonest symptom of laryngeal disease is hoarseness or change in the normal voice, and if this persists for more than two weeks after medical treatment the larynx must be examined. Other indications include stridor and examination of the movements of the vocal cords in patients before thyroidectomy. In patients with dysphagia examination of the larynx may disclose a postcricoid carcinoma, and earache may be a result of referred pain from a carcinoma in the laryngeal area.

Treatment—Simple lesions such as cysts and vocal-cord nodules may be removed with special instruments by using the method of direct laryngoscopy, and biopsy of a suspicious lesion in the larynx is an important procedure. It must be remembered that treatment of early carcinoma of the vocal cords is curative.

Contraindications to laryngoscopy—Contraindications are few, but the procedure cannot be performed in acute inflammations of the throat that give rise to trismus—for example, a peritonsillar abscess. Direct laryngoscopy is inadvisable in acute epiglottitis, as it could lead to a spread of inflammatory oedema to the glottis.

Indirect laryngoscopy

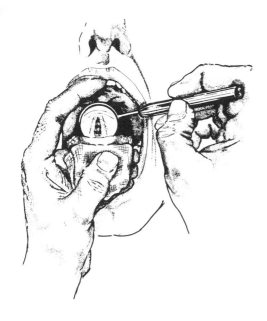

This is the method of examining the larynx from above with a laryngeal mirror. It is a simple procedure that is within the capabilities of every doctor who is willing to practise, and should be performed more often than it is.

Instruments—A laryngeal mirror or mirrors and a spirit lamp, or hot water if a spirit lamp is not available; gauze swabs for holding the tongue; and a light source, which may be a battery-operated head lamp or a head mirror using reflected light that may come from an electric bulb or a good torch.

Procedure—The patient is seated in front of the examiner, who sits at about the same height. The light is directed on to the lips of the patient, who is asked to open his mouth and protrude his tongue as far as possible. The tongue is grasped between the thumb and middle fingers of the examiner's left hand through the gauze swab. It is important not to pull the tongue too far forward or the frenum will impinge on the lower teeth and cause pain. The index finger of the left hand is rested on the upper teeth to steady the hand.

The mirror is warmed over the spirit lamp, the flame being directed on to the glass surface. After the temperature has been tested on the examiner's cheek the mirror, held in the right hand, is introduced into the mouth and placed at the back of the uvula without touching the tongue, as this would smear the surface of the mirror. Steady pressure is maintained on the soft palate, and the light is directed on to the mirror. A reflection of the interior of the larynx will be seen, and the various structures may be examined in sequence by tilting the mirror.

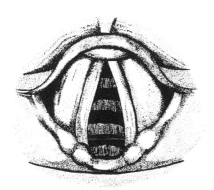

The base of the tongue, epiglottis, valleculae, aryepiglottic folds, false cords, true cords, and upper tracheal rings can all be seen in turn. The mobility of the cords can be tested by asking the patient to say "ee," when the glottis should close. The mirror may have to be removed and warmed again and the examination repeated before the full information is obtained.

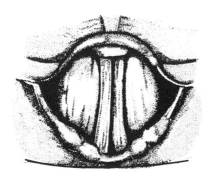

Difficulties of indirect laryngoscopy—Some patients have an overactive "gag" reflex, and examination is difficult unless the soft palate is sprayed with an anaesthetic solution such as 5% cocaine or an amethocaine lozenge is sucked before the examination. It is difficult to examine children by indirect laryngoscopy, but sometimes the larynx may be seen by placing the mirror almost horizontally against the hard palate instead of the soft palate, so that the gag reflex is not excited. The anterior commissure of the larynx is the most difficult part to see, and complete examination of the piriform fossae is not possible by indirect laryngoscopy.

It should be remembered that the structures of the larynx are seen in a mirror, so that the anterior part points away from the examiner and the right-hand structures are seen on the left.

5% Cocaine solution
or
Amethocaine lozenge

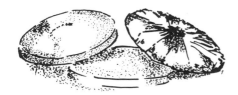

Laryngoscopy

Direct laryngoscopy

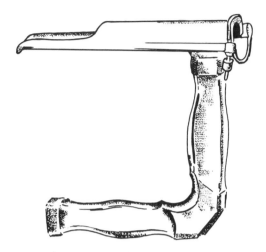

In direct laryngoscopy the larynx is looked at from above through a tube with an integral light source; there is no distortion or shortening of the structures, as occurs when a mirror is used, and the image is not reversed.

Surgical instruments may be passed down the laryngoscope and limited surgery carried out, and accurate biopsy is possible. It is the method of choice in children.

Contraindications—Contraindications are few and would include injuries and disease of the cervical spine; severe trismus; and appreciable laryngeal obstruction, when a tracheostomy should be done first.

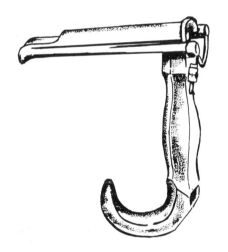

Method—Under general anaesthesia with a hard, narrow-bore catheter inserted through the mouth into the trachea the patient rests on his back with his head flexed against his neck and his teeth protected by a guard. When the muscles are relaxed the laryngoscope is inserted, and the structures in the vicinity of the larynx and the larynx itself are inspected so that all the structures are seen. The laryngoscope can be fixed in position by suspension attachments to the chest of the patient or the head of the operating table, allowing the surgeon two hands to perform endolaryngeal surgery.

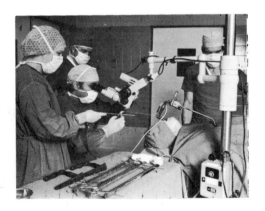

Microlaryngoscopy—This method was first described by Kleinsasser in 1968. A special wide laryngoscope is used, held in position by a suspension system. The larynx is examined with the Zeiss operating microscope, which gives a magnified binocular view of the larynx. Fine instruments are available for accurate surgical treatment of such lesions as polyps, singers' nodes, etc, and accurate biopsy of suspicious lesions is possible. This is now the method of choice for treating lesions of the larynx endoscopically.

Complications of direct laryngoscopy—These are few and include damage to the teeth and laceration of the lips and pharyngeal wall.

The photograph of the larynx is reproduced by courtesy of Mr T R Bull.

TAPPING ASCITES

E RYAN   G NEALE

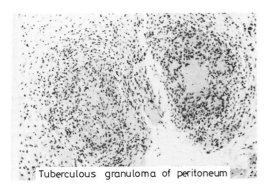

Tuberculous granuloma of peritoneum

Tapping ascites is a simple, safe procedure for which the indications are as follows: (1) to investigate the cause of ascites and when necessary take a specimen of peritoneum for biopsy; (2) to assess bacterial infection of ascitic fluid; and (3) to treat by (*a*) removing fluid to relieve abdominal discomfort or severe dyspnoea or (*b*) introducing chemotherapeutic agents.

Tapping the abdomen is used principally as an aid to diagnosis. With modern drugs fluid rarely has to be removed from the peritoneal cavity to relieve severe dyspnoea or the pain of abdominal distention. Occasionally, in a patient with liver disease, fluid may be removed from the abdomen, ultrafiltered, and reinfused into a systemic vein as an adjunct to treatment with diuretics.

Detecting ascites

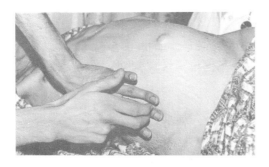

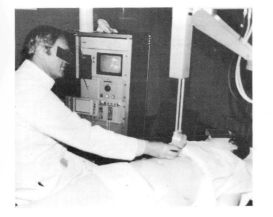

The clinical signs of fullness in the flanks, shifting dullness, and a fluid wave require the presence of at least 500 ml of free fluid. If the patient can get on to his hands and knees smaller volumes of fluid gravitating to the periumbilical area may be detected, thereby allowing the "puddle" sign to be elicited. Ascites may be diagnosed when none exists, especially in patients who have fluid-filled viscera (for example, fluid in loops of small intestine or in large, lax ovarian cysts), and, conversely, may not be detected when it is localised by peritoneal attachments.

Ultrasound appears to be the most useful investigation in detecting small quantities of fluid especially when these are localised. Table I shows the principal causes of free fluid in the abdomen.

TABLE I—*Causes of ascites*

Associated with chronic disorders	*Associated with acute abdomen*
Common causes:	Bacterial peritonitis
Cirrhosis of the liver	Trauma (haemoperitoneum)
Abdominal cancer	Acute pancreatitis
Tuberculous peritonitis	Strangulated viscera (especially intestine)
Heart disease (especially constrictive pericarditis)	
Rare causes:	*In the neonate* (*extremely rare*)
Liver disease without cirrhosis	Renal abnormality (with leakage of urine)
Hepatic vein occlusion	Intestinal abnormality (for example, obstruction
Severe hepatitis	with perforation)
Chronic pancreatic disease	Cardiac failure
Myxoedema	Cirrhosis
Chronic renal disease	Infection (for example, toxoplasmosis)
Polyserositis (for example, systemic lupus	
erythematosus)	
Other inflammatory conditions (for example,	
Crohn's disease)	
Ovarian disease	

Tapping ascites

Precautions

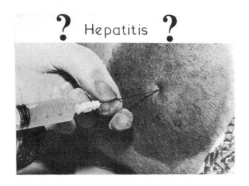

Provided sterile methods are used and a few precautions taken, passing a fine needle into the peritoneal cavity is totally safe even when fluid cannot be aspirated. The removal of large quantities of fluid is rarely necessary and may lead to hypovolaemia and, consequently, to oliguria and hyponatraemia. Special care must be taken in handling instruments and aspirated fluid when treating patients who have viral hepatitis or in whom there is circulating hepatitis B antigen.

Procedure

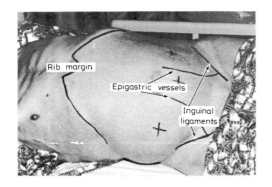

Explain the procedure to the patient and get him to empty his bladder. Ask him to lie relaxed in a supine position. Re-examine the abdomen and select a site for puncture. (Usually this site will be in an area in which there is shifting dullness and under which there appear to be no solid organs. The iliac fossae, away from the inferior epigastric blood vessels and scars, are the areas most often used, and it may be helpful for the patient to roll slightly to the side of the operation in order to maximise the area of dullness. Aspiration through the less-vascular linea alba is occasionally used for therapeutic procedures and before laparoscopy.)

Put on a mask and sterile gloves. Clean the skin and infiltrate 3-6 ml of local anaesthetic into the anterior abdominal wall down to the parietal peritoneum. Attach a long fine needle (19-23 gauge) to a large syringe and introduce the needle into the abdominal cavity. (Often a sense of give is felt in passing across the anterior and posterior fascial layers and, to a less extent, in perforating the peritoneum.) Aspirate gently. Fluid will flow easily into the syringe if the tip of the needle is correctly placed. If no fluid is obtained reposition either the patient or the needle. Remove up to 50 ml of fluid, withdraw the needle, and apply a simple dressing to the skin. In patients with suspected tuberculosis it is worth while taking much larger quantities of fluid and using the centrifuged deposit to isolate the causative organism.

Aftercare and complications

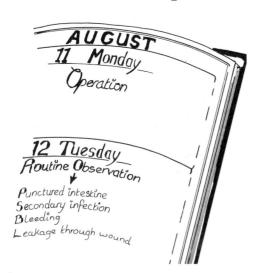

Tapping ascites rarely leads to complications. Inadvertent puncture of the intestine is rare, and even if intestinal contents are aspirated secondary infection is most unusual. Routine observation for 24-28 hours is sufficient aftercare to detect the exceptionally rare complications of bleeding or infection. Scrotal oedema has been described after paracentesis, especially when tapping of ascites is associated with laparoscopy: it responds to simple management.

In patients with malignant ascites persistent leakage through puncture wounds is sometimes a problem. For this reason incisions in the abdominal wall should be kept as small as possible and sufficient fluid should be removed to reduce the pressure in the abdominal cavity.

Specimens

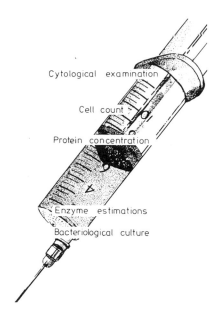

Cytological examination

Cell count

Protein concentration

Enzyme estimations

Bacteriological culture

The appearance of the fluid removed by tapping the abdomen should be noted. A cloudy fluid often means peritonitis; uniform bloodstaining is most often found in patients who have cancer or who have suffered trauma to the abdomen; and a milky fluid indicates chylous ascites.

Aliquots of the fluid are sent to the laboratory for cytological examination, cell count, measurement of protein concentration, and, in selected cases, enzyme estimations and bacteriological culture. Table II summarises the results to be expected, but these must be interpreted cautiously.

Fluid is removed from the peritoneal cavity most often in patients with ascites due to cirrhosis, especially when a complication is suspected. Spontaneous bacterial infection is a frequent worry, and thus abdominal tap should be performed in any patient with cirrhosis and ascites if he develops fever without obvious cause, abdominal pain, diarrhoea, or encephalopathy. In uncomplicated cases the fluid from a patient with cirrhosis is clear and yellow, contains few white cells, and has a low concentration of total protein. A high white cell count may indicate spontaneous bacterial peritonitis; a high protein concentration may point to hepatoma; and high amylase activity is associated with pancreatic disease. Nevertheless, 10% of patients with ascites secondary to uncomplicated cirrhosis have white cell counts of over $1 \times 10^9/l$ (1000/mm³), and high protein concentrations have been described in a similar proportion.

TABLE II—*Guide to results of laboratory tests on ascitic fluid*

Source of ascites	Appearance	Protein concentration (g/l)	Total white cell count ($\times 10^9$/l)	Polymorphonuclear leucocytes (%)	Lymphocytes (%)	Amylase activity	Microscopy	Culture
Uncomplicated cirrhosis	Clear	<30 (occasionally high)	<0·3 (occasionally high)	<25	>75	Low	Negative	Negative
Neoplastic	Bloodstained or clear	>25 (sometimes low)	0·1-1·0	<50	>50	Low	May be positive	Negative
Pancreatic	Clear or serosanguinous	>30	Variable	Variable	Variable	High	Negative	Negative
Tuberculous	Clear-cloudy	>30	Variable	<50	>50	Low	Positive peritoneal biopsy	Positive
Nephrotic	Clear	<10	<0·3	<25	>75	Low	Negative	Negative
Cardiac	Clear	Variable (sometimes high)	<0·3	<25	>75	Low	Negative	Negative
Spontaneous bacterial peritonitis	Cloudy	>25	>0·3	>75	<25	Low	Positive	Positive

Therapeutic implications

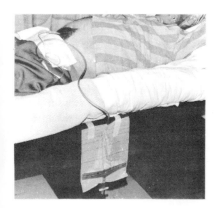

Occasionally in patients with massive ascites a large quantity of fluid may have to be removed. This may best be performed through the avascular linea alba. Anaesthetise and cleanse the abdominal wall and pass a plastic intravenous cannula (14 gauge) through it. Remove the introducer and thread the cannula into the abdomen until fluid flows freely. Connect the cannula to a drainage bag and control the flow of fluid with an adjustable clip. Remove up to two litres over about four hours (rapid removal of fluid may cause hypotension). If necessary reposition the patient or the cannula to maintain the flow of fluid. Cytotoxic agents may be introduced through the cannula in appropriate dosage. After sufficient fluid has been removed take out the cannula and apply a firm dressing.

Tapping ascites

Peritoneal biopsy

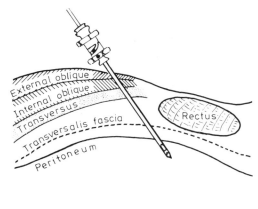

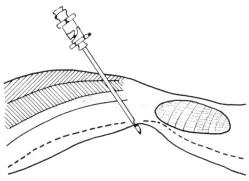

Indication—Biopsy of the peritoneum is useful in diagnosing non-purulent ascites in which the fluid has a protein concentration of over 25 g/l, is not rich in amylase, and in which direct examination does not show malignant cells or acid-fast bacilli.

Method—Ascertain the presence of ascitic fluid by tapping the abdomen in the standard manner. Remove the exploring needle and introduce an Abrams punch through a small skin incision. Attach the punch to a syringe and open the notch by twisting the hexagonal grip anticlockwise. Aspirate a little fluid. Angle the open notch against the peritoneal surface and withdraw the punch slowly until it engages the abdominal wall. Twist the hexagonal grip clockwise and withdraw the punch. Remove any tissue from the edge of the notch and, if necessary, repeat the procedure (it is virtually impossible to obtain tissue when the peritoneal surface is normal).

Specimens—Routine histological procedures are used to examine the specimens obtained. Peritoneal biopsy gives a high yield in patients with tuberculous peritonitis and is also useful in diagnosing cancer seedlings affecting the parietal peritoneum.

Tapping the acute abdomen

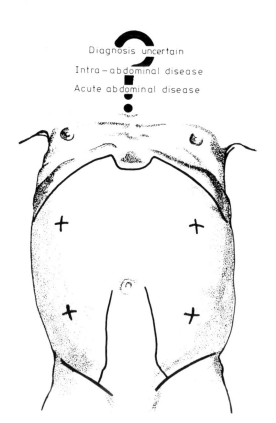

Paracentesis is not used universally to investigate patients with acute abdominal disorders even though many reports over the past 50 years have extolled its value. It is used when the diagnosis is in doubt, especially after abdominal trauma. The method is similar to that used in tapping a clinically demonstrable volume of ascitic fluid, but the site of puncture is determined by the local clinical findings. If there is generalised abdominal tenderness tapping in the four quadrants of the abdomen may be performed followed by needling the flanks. Local anaesthesia is usually unnecessary for this procedure. If the tap yields no fluid and there is still doubt about the diagnosis it may be worth while attempting to aspirate fluid from the pouch of Douglas. This is done by inserting a dialysis catheter through the linea alba, and some doctors believe that peritoneal lavage using this technique may be helpful.

Indications for the procedure are as follows: (1) puzzling diagnostic problems, especially in those regarded as presenting high operative risks; (2) obtunded patients in whom there are signs suggesting intra-abdominal disease (especially after trauma); and (3) suspected non-surgical acute abdominal disease (for example, pancreatitis).

Contraindications—Paracentesis should not be carried out on: (1) patients in whom the diagnosis appears to be clear-cut or in whom a diagnosis may be achieved by non-invasive investigations; (2) patients with multiple scars and distended bowel; (3) patients with localised inflammatory disease (results are usually unhelpful); and (4) pregnant patients.

Precautions—Analysis of fluid obtained by lavage should not be relied on if the results are inconsistent with other findings. The procedure is probably most usefully performed if one doctor in the hospital takes special responsibility for the investigation and its interpretation.

PROCTOSCOPY AND SIGMOIDOSCOPY

D J ELLIS   P G BEVAN

Uses

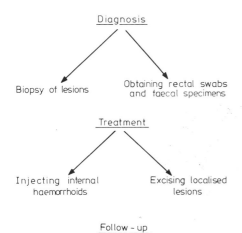

Both proctoscopy and sigmoidoscopy are used for diagnosis, treatment, and follow-up. Lesions of the anal canal and rectum and lower sigmoid colon can be diagnosed and biopsy carried out. Rectal swabs are sent for bacteriological studies or specimens of faeces for identification of parasites. Internal haemorrhoids can be treated by injection through a proctoscope and excision or diathermy of small localised lesions carried out through a sigmoidoscope. Follow-up examinations are useful to show whether inflammatory conditions are subsiding, persisting, or worsening. The response to medical treatment can be monitored—for example, improvement in non-specific proctitis after a course of steroid enemas.

Indications

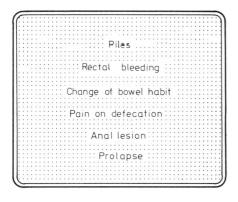

Proctoscopy or sigmoidoscopy, or both, should be carried out on all patients who complain of the following symptoms: piles; rectal bleeding; change of bowel habit, especially recurring attacks of diarrhoea; pain or difficulty in defecation; lesions around the anal opening (abscesses, fistulae, discharge, ulcers, external piles, pruritus); and prolapse.

Preparation

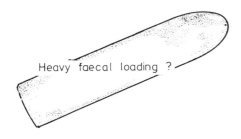

Pre-examination bowel preparation is generally unnecessary and may disguise abnormalities by producing oedema of the rectal and colonic mucosa. It may, however, be necessary in patients with heavy faecal loading of the distal colon and rectum. A normal bowel action should be encouraged on the morning of the examination.

Proctoscopy and sigmoidoscopy

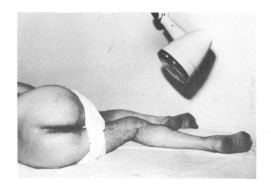

Proctoscopy can be done without difficulty or discomfort in the doctor's surgery or outpatient clinic without general anaesthesia. It is important to ensure that the patient is lying in the correct position and is comfortable and relaxed. The left lateral position is usually advocated, with the bottom pushed backwards and both hips flexed, the right leg above the left to tilt the anal opening upwards. In obese patients it is helpful to place a cushion under the buttocks.

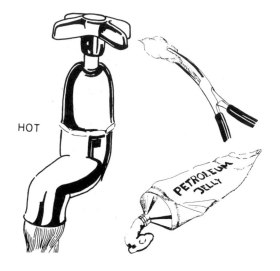

HOT

PETROLEUM JELLY

The first step is to separate the buttocks and inspect the anal verge carefully for pruritus, external piles, a fissure, or a fistula. It is essential to insert the lubricated forefinger through the anal canal and examine the lower part of the rectum before attempting to pass a proctoscope or sigmoidoscope. Anal stenosis or severe pain on digital examination is a contraindication to the passage of either instrument.

The calibre of the anal canal should be judged at the preliminary examination with the index finger, and too large an instrument should not be used. An adequate source of light must be available before the proctoscope is inserted—this may be a bright torch or Anglepoise lamp, or a side bulb built into the proctoscope. A straight pair of artery forceps should be at hand holding a pledget of damp cotton-wool to clean the mucosal surface or remove faecal matter through the proctoscope. The proctoscope should first be warmed under the hot tap, dried, and well lubricated. It is passed by pushing the head of the obturator firmly but gently through the anal canal in the direction of the umbilicus, and when through the anus it is turned in the direction of the patient's head and inserted to the hilt. The obturator must be kept fully engaged in the proctoscope during insertion to avoid nipping the anal mucosa. Close inspection is made as the instrument is withdrawn, firstly of the lower rectal mucosa and then of the anal canal, noting any haemorrhoids bulging into the lumen of the proctoscope or the linear raw area of a fissure.

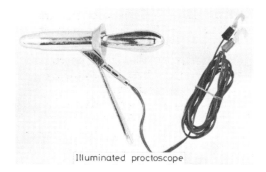

Illuminated proctoscope

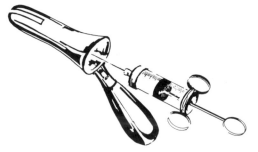

Injecting internal haemorrhoids—An injecting proctoscope is used for this procedure and rotated so as to allow the pile to bulge into the side aperture. Through a special haemorrhoid needle 3-5 ml of 5% phenol in oil is injected submucously into the base of the pile; the injection must not be intravascular.

Sigmoidoscopy

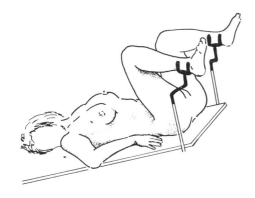

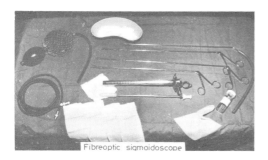

Fibreoptic sigmoidoscope

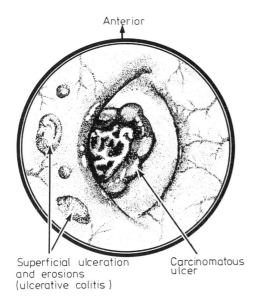

Superficial ulceration and erosions (ulcerative colitis)

Carcinomatous ulcer

Complete visualisation of the rectum and lower sigmoid colon usually needs a general anaesthetic. This is a good rule for the learner, but with increasing experience and confidence general anaesthesia may be omitted in most cases. The lithotomy position is most commonly used, with a head-down tilt to the table. The lower abdomen should first be palpated for the presence of a mass; digital palpation of the rectum then follows, and finally bimanual palpation with the right index finger in the rectum and the left hand on the lower abdomen. The prone jack-knife position has its advocates but precludes abdominal palpation. Sigmoidoscopy can be done without a general anaesthetic in the left lateral position, and a transparent disposable plastic sigmoidoscope is probably the best and most comfortable instrument for this, although passing the rectosigmoid bend may be so painful as to be impossible. The traditional sigmoidoscope has a proximal bulb light, but the newer fibreoptic model with a circular distal light is to be preferred. The insufflating bulb is an important part of the instrument, as the upper half of the rectum and lower sigmoid can be seen clearly only when air is blown in to distend the lumen. A long alligator biopsy forceps should be available and also a long pledget-holding forceps for cleaning the mucosa.

As soon as the end of the sigmoidoscope has penetrated the anal canal the obturator is removed, the inspecting end closed, and examination of the rectal mucosa carried out carefully from below upwards. When the upper rectum is reached the end of the sigmoidoscope is moved to the patient's left, backwards, and then forwards to round the rectosigmoid bend into the lower sigmoid colon. It is vital to get a clear view of this area, as it cannot be felt digitally per rectum or by lower abdominal palpation. The operator must be prepared patiently to clear the rectum of faeces by digital removal, scooping them out in the sigmoidoscope or using pledgets on long-handled forceps. A sucker must always be available but used gently and its end guarded with a rubber tube. The instrument must never be forced upwards, and blanching of the mucosa is a danger sign.

The mucous membrane is inspected for colour, texture, and mobility. Erosions, ulcers, adenomas, polyps, and the raised edge of a carcinoma are looked for and biopsy specimens taken. The barrel of the sigmoidoscope is calibrated in centimetres, and the distance of any lesion from the anal verge must be noted. Rectal biopsy specimens should normally be taken posteriorly 6-8 cm from the anal verge; high anterior biopsies run the risk of perforation. The presence of blood and pus in the lumen should be noted and also the colour, consistency, and shape of the faecal masses— for example, diverticular disease can be diagnosed by finding a contracted corrugated faecal cast. Proctoscopy should be done after sigmoidoscopy, as anal lesions may be missed through the sigmoidoscope.

Final steps

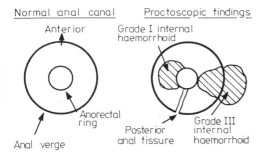

Normal anal canal

Anterior

Anorectal ring

Anal verge

Proctoscopic findings

Grade I internal haemorrhoid

Posterior anal fissure

Grade III internal haemorrhoid

If stretching of the anal canal needs to be carried out for anal stenosis this should be done after sigmoidoscopy (but before proctoscopy). All findings must be noted carefully, and this is usually done in diagrammatic form.

PERCUTANEOUS CENTRAL VENOUS CANNULATION

M ROSEN,   I P LATTO   W SHANG NG

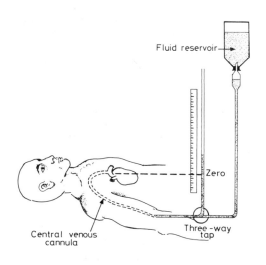

Central venous cannulation in surgical practice and intensive care has become more common with the impetus derived from experience in cardiac surgery and developments in disposable plastic catheters and cannulae. The procedure may, however, result in serious hazard and even death. There are numerous approaches to the central veins, and the methods and equipment described here have been chosen as those most likely to be safe and successful in the hands of an inexperienced houseman called on to cannulate an adult either breathing spontaneously or receiving lung ventilation.

Indications and contraindications

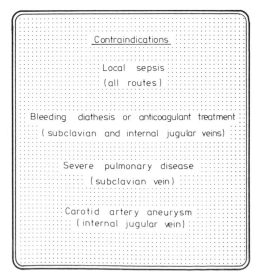

Contraindications

Local sepsis
(all routes)

Bleeding diathesis or anticoagulant treatment
(subclavian and internal jugular veins)

Severe pulmonary disease
(subclavian vein)

Carotid artery aneurysm
(internal jugular vein)

Central venous pressure is the resultant of venous blood volume, right ventricular function, and venous tone. Rapid changes in blood volume, especially associated with impaired right heart function, are the most common reason for monitoring central venous pressure. Peripheral venous pressures do not reflect these changes reliably. In an emergency only a central vein may be accessible for administration of a rapid life-saving infusion. This route is also widely used for long-term intravenous alimentation.

There are no contraindications to the method per se. Venepuncture should be avoided, however, at any site at which there is sepsis. Apical emphysema or bullae contraindicate infraclavicular or supraclavicular approaches to the subclavian vein. A carotid artery aneurysm precludes using the internal jugular vein on the same side. Furthermore, it may be wise to reconsider central venous cannulation in hypocoagulation and hypercoagulation states or if there is septicaemia.

Procedure

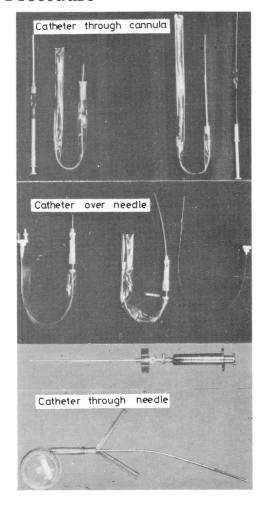

Sterility—Sterility should be maintained during the insertion of the cannula. The skin should be carefully cleaned—for example, with 0·5% chlorhexidine in 70% alcohol—and sterile towels applied round the site. The operator should wear a mask, gown, and gloves, and in an emergency gloves at least should be worn. Although some catheter systems are designed to be used ungloved, in practice contamination may sometimes occur through an error or technical difficulty.

Equipment—(1) Catheter through cannula. A cannula on the outside of a needle is placed in the vein and the needle withdrawn. A catheter, previously checked to match the internal diameter of the cannula, is then threaded into the vein. When the catheter is in position the cannula is withdrawn. If the catheter has no stylet dissecting forceps may be necessary to feed it forward. (2) Catheter over needle. In an arm vein the needle and catheter are placed in the vein, the needle (which is attached to a wire) withdrawn, and the catheter advanced into position. Long needles and cannulae (100 mm) are available for use in the internal jugular and subclavian veins. (3) Catheter through needle. This is the simplest method and still widely used. It has been condemned because improper use may result in the catheter being sheared off. The needle is inserted in the vein and the catheter then advanced slowly by threading it forward or unwinding it if it is coiled on a drum, avoiding force if any obstruction to progress is felt. Only after the needle is withdrawn should the catheter be pulled back, always by gripping it beyond the needle tip and never by pulling it through the needle. (4) Catheter over guide wire. A flexible guide wire is inserted into the vein through a needle. After removal of the needle the catheter is inserted over the wire, which guides it into the vein.

A stylet is useful to thread the catheter forward and to indicate the length of catheter in the patient. The presumptive position of the tip can be estimated and the catheter withdrawn so that the tip lies above the nipple line. A precoiled catheter (the drum) can be more frequently placed in the superior vena cava.

Methods

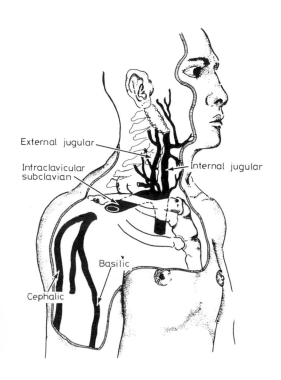

The techniques are described in order of safety and effectiveness. In each, air embolism is avoided by maintaining the venous pressure above atmospheric by position or a tourniquet on the limb. If the patient is conscious the skin should be infiltrated with a local anaesthetic using a fine needle.

Arm veins—The median (basilic) arm veins are the safest approach to the central venous system. The cephalic vein curves sharply to join the axillary vein through the deep fascia at the shoulder, which may impede passage of a catheter. This results in less successful central placement, but it is still worth attempting. The veins are distended by a tourniquet. The head is turned to the same side to compress the neck veins, and the arm is abducted. The catheter should be of 600 mm minimum length. When the tourniquet is released air embolism may occur, so depress the proximal end of the catheter below the level of the patient's elbow.

External jugular vein—The external jugular vein runs from the angle of the mandible to behind the middle of the clavicle and joins the subclavian vein. The patient is placed in a 20° head-down position with the head turned to the opposite side. The most prominent vein is chosen. If neither vein becomes visible or palpable cannulation is inadvisable. In about half the attempts the catheter cannot be threaded into an intrathoracic vein, but successful central placement may be helped by digital pressure above the clavicle, by depressing the shoulder, or by flushing through the catheter. The use of a Seldinger wire or a spinal J-shaped wire increases the incidence of successful central placement of the catheter. The use of excessive force should be avoided. Satisfactory measurement of central venous pressure is sometimes possible from the external jugular vein or from the junction of the external jugular and subclavian veins. This junction is a common site for the distal tip when the catheter will not thread centrally.

Percutaneous central venous cannulation

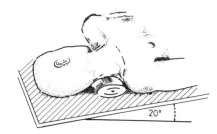

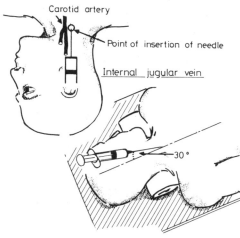

Carotid artery

Point of insertion of needle

Internal jugular vein

Internal jugular vein—The internal jugular veins run behind the sternomastoid close to the lateral border of the carotid artery. The vein may be cannulated with a low incidence of major complications by an approach well above the clavicle. The patient is placed in a 20° head-down position with the head turned to the opposite side. The right side is preferred to avoid injury to the thoracic duct and is also easier for the right-handed operator. The sternomastoid muscle, cricoid cartilage, and carotid artery are identified. With the other hand the carotid artery is palpated and protected at the level of the cricoid cartilage. The needle is attached to a saline-filled syringe and inserted just lateral to the artery. The needle is directed towards the feet parallel to the midline with the syringe raised 30° above the skin. Gentle aspiration is maintained as the needle is advanced. A flush of blood into the syringe signifies entry into the vein. If the artery is punctured use firm compression for five minutes.

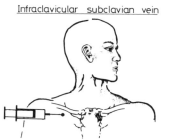

Infraclavicular subclavian vein

Infraclavicular subclavian vein—The subclavian vein is particularly suitable for administering long-term parenteral nutrition. It is widely patent even in states of circulatory collapse, so that subclavian venepuncture may be the only route for rapid infusion. Puncture and catheterisation of the subclavian vein is a blind procedure. Serious harm can be inflicted on nearby vital structures, and deaths have been reported. The most common complication is pneumothorax. The procedure, therefore, should not ordinarily be performed by an inexperienced operator without close supervision. The subclavian vein lies in the angle formed by the medial one-third of the clavicle and the first rib, in which the subclavian vein crosses over the first rib to enter the thoracic cavity. There is some variation in the anatomy of this region, which has prompted the use of an ultrasound probe to facilitate locating the position of the subclavian vein. This manoeuvre, however, is unlikely to reduce the incidence of pneumothorax. The patient rests supine, tilted 20° head down. Either side may be used, although the right side is preferable. The patient's head is turned to the opposite side. The midpoint of the clavicle and the suprasternal notch should be identified. The distance between the skin puncture and the vein necessitates using a long needle and cannula. The needle is attached to a saline-filled syringe and inserted below the lower border of the midpoint of the clavicle. The needle tip is advanced close to the undersurface of the clavicle, aiming at the suprasternal notch. While the needle is advanced gentle aspiration should be maintained, and a flush of blood indicates that the vein is entered. If the attempt is unsuccessful, further attempts may be made, altering the direction of the needle only when it has been withdrawn to just beneath the skin. A chest radiograph should always be taken to check for pneumothorax.

Diameters of needles or cannulae and lengths of catheters recommended for each route of insertion

Route of insertion	Outside diameter of needle or cannula	Minimum length of catheter (mm)
Arm vein	14G	600
External jugular vein	16 or 14G	200
Internal jugular vein	14G	150*
Subclavian vein	14G	150*

*Long cannulae are available.

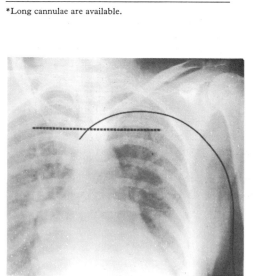

Checking and testing—Blood should be aspirated to ensure that the catheter is in a vascular space before injecting fluid. If the line is connected to a bottle of fluid that is lowered below the patient blood should flow freely under the influence of gravity. On connection to a column of fluid for measurements of central venous pressure the fluid column should show slow oscillations related to respiration and quicker oscillations related to the heart beats. A chest radiograph should be taken to confirm that the position of the tip is above the right atrium, preferably not more than 2 cm below a line joining the lower borders of the clavicles.

Management

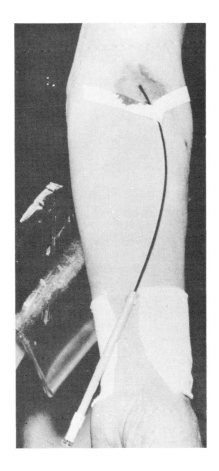

Fixing the catheter—Once satisfactorily placed, the catheter should be fixed carefully to prevent inadvertent withdrawal or movement further into the vein. Firm fixation probably also reduces the incidence of thrombophlebitis. Adhesive tape (1 cm width) is crossed over to grip the catheter firmly, away from the venepuncture site. An alternative, especially for longer-term use, is to secure the catheter with a skin suture.

Asepsis—The most scrupulous attention to detail is needed to keep venous catheters infection free. Strict aseptic technique during the insertion of the catheter is mandatory. For long-term parenteral nutrition the site where the catheter enters the skin may be led away from the vein by creating a subcutaneous tunnel. Additions to intravenous fluids should preferably be introduced in the aseptic laboratory of the pharmacy. The intravenous giving set should be changed daily, an aseptic technique being used while connecting it to the catheter. Injecting drugs into the venous catheter and taking blood samples through stopcocks should be avoided if possible. Regular bacteriological monitoring of the venepuncture site should be carried out. It is important to be vigilant to detect catheter-related infections. If an infection occurs the catheter should be removed immediately.

Clotting—It is important to maintain flow through the catheter to prevent reflux of blood and clotting. After taking intermittent measurements of venous pressure it is a common fault to forget to turn on the infusion again, resulting in a catheter blocked by clot. The catheter must then be replaced.

Complications

IMMEDIATE
Arterial puncture
Pneumothorax
Cardiac arrhythmias
Injury to thoracic duct
Injury to nerves

IMMEDIATE OR LATER
Air embolism
Catheter embolus

LATER
Myocardial perforation and tamponade
Hydrothorax
Infection
Venous thrombosis

Complications of central venous catheterisation mostly fall into two categories—firstly, those that occur at the time of catheterisation and result from injury to some vital structure; and, secondly, those that occur at a later stage and are associated with catheter-related thrombophlebitis and infection. In addition to these two groups air embolism, catheter embolism, cardiac arrhythmias, and perforation of the myocardium may occur at any time. When arm or external jugular veins are used serious immediate complications are rare. The veins are usually visible and palpable. Catheters lying in peripheral veins, however, often lead to thrombophlebitis if left in position for more than one or two days. Most immediate and serious complications are a feature of blind venepuncture of the subclavian and, to a less extent, internal jugular veins. Injury to many structures related to the thoracic inlet has been reported: pneumothorax, haemothorax, arterial puncture, and damage to the thoracic duct and phrenic nerve. The complication rates reported after catheterisation of the deep veins range between zero and 15% and are probably dependent on the experience of the operator.

ASPIRATION AND INJECTION OF JOINTS

PETER WILLIAMS   MICHAEL GUMPEL

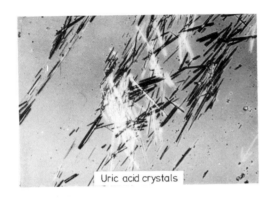

Uric acid crystals

Therapeutic injection of joints and periarticular structures is simple: the ability to perform this procedure as primary care may save the patient needless waiting for hospital appointments. Examination of synovial fluid for diagnostic purposes in patients with unexplained or acute synovitis may be vital: familiarity with the technique will increase the likelihood of obtaining such fluid.

Indications

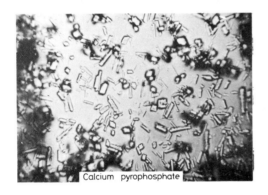

Calcium pyrophosphate

(1) Diagnostic aspiration in cases of suspected septic arthritis, crystal-induced synovitis, and haemarthrosis.

(2) Therapeutic aspiration for tense effusions, septic effusions, and haemarthrosis.

(3) Therapeutic injections of corticosteroids for persistent localised synovitis or soft-tissue lesions.

(4) Introduction of contrast media for diagnostic arthrography.

Cautionary considerations

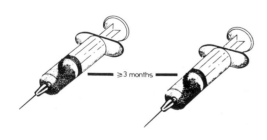

≥3 months

Frequent use of steroid injections in weight-bearing joints, particularly in osteoarthrosis, is not recommended, and the interval between injections should not normally be less than three months. The patient should be warned not to be overenthusiastic in using the joint in the 24 hours after injection.

If septic arthritis is possible or the joint fluid is purulent, steroids should not be injected until negative bacterial cultures have been obtained. The possibility of tuberculosis as a cause of "synovitis" should be considered, particularly in immigrants.

Iatrogenic infection is rare with disposable syringes and needles, and the risk is minimised by a careful sterile technique. The patient should nevertheless be warned to seek medical advice for increased pain or swelling after intra-articular injections. Certain soft-tissue injections, particularly for tennis elbow and painful arc shoulder, may cause increased pain for a day or two afterwards, and the patient should be warned of this before injection.

Materials for injection

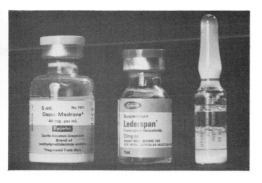

Use lignocaine or Xylocaine (without adrenaline) 1-2%. We usually use hydrocortisone acetate injection and reserve the longer-acting, more expensive preparations (for example, methylprednisolone acetate and triamcinolone (hex) acetonide) for patients in whom hydrocortisone acetate is only briefly effective or for small joints. Because of the risk of atrophy of the skin and subcutaneous tissues hydrocortisone acetate is preferable for soft-tissue injection. Multidose containers should be used only if you are the sole user.

General procedure

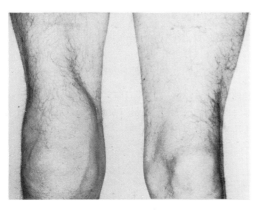

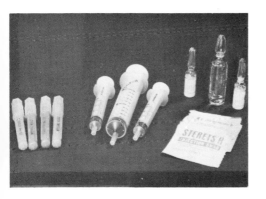

Diagnostic aspiration or injection is much easier when appreciable swelling is present, as less precision is required in placing the needle. Before starting, carefully feel the bony margins of the joint space. Use the thumbnail to mark the joint space, and if in doubt move one bone so that you can feel its movement on one side of the joint. Check that you have easily available all you need: choice of needles and syringes, local anaesthetic (or saline), requisite specimen containers, and, for large effusions, a jug or basin nearby. For aspiration followed by injection draw up the steroid beforehand and make sure the needles are not too tightly jammed on the syringes.

Prepare the skin carefully with chlorhexidine in 5% spirit or surgical spirit—not Savlon. A rigorous no-touch technique is for the experienced and for simple injections; sterile gloves, a sterile pack, and a generous area of prepared skin for the less experienced. With experience it is rarely necessary to use local anaesthetic, and a subcutaneous bleb is usually sufficient. Local anaesthetic in the syringe is useful when difficulty in entering the joint is expected or to clear the needle and check that there is free and easy flow once the joint is entered.

In joint aspiration the needle size is important. For thick, purulent or chronic effusions a white (19-gauge) needle is usually needed, otherwise a green one (21) will suffice. For finger and toe joints use a blue (23) needle, which is usually used for injecting small quantities.

When effusions are purulent send specimens for microbiological examination and measurement of protein and glucose concentrations (in a small fluoride container), and a heparinised sample for cytology and crystal examination. Identifying crystals requires some experience, and at night it may be best to keep a sample refrigerated to be re-examined the next morning.

Ankle joint

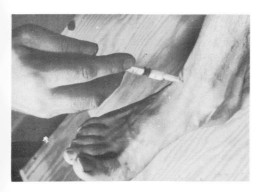

With the foot slightly plantar flexed, palpate the joint line anteriorly between the tendons of extensor hallucis longus laterally and tibialis anterior medially just above the tip of the medial malleolus. Direct the needle slightly sideways, backwards, and upwards. Fluid may be aspirated if there is an effusion. Hydrocortisone acetate 25 mg is appropriate.

Aspiration and injection of joints

Knee

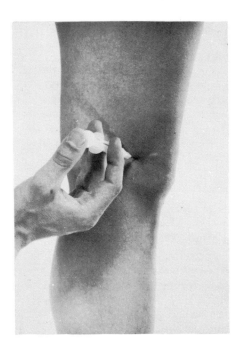

The patient should be as comfortable as possible, lying down with sufficient pillows. The knee may be slightly flexed and muscles relaxed. Palpate the posterior edge of the patella medially or laterally and move the patella gently sideways to feel the femoral surfaces below. The patient should be sufficiently relaxed that the patella can be moved freely; otherwise, aspiration is virtually impossible. Maintain a gentle conversation rather than grim silence. Insert the needle horizontally or slightly downwards into the joint in the gap between patella and femur; once behind the patella it must be within the joint. A slight resistance may often be felt as the needle goes through the synovial membrane. If no fluid can be aspirated check that the patient's quadriceps muscle is relaxed and that the needle is not blocked by injecting local anaesthetic. If this flows freely the needle is intra-articular. One last trick is to rotate the needle, as a synovial villus or fibrin body may be against the bevel.

Small effusions may sometimes be found in the medial or lateral pouches, and fluid will appear in the syringe as the needle is withdrawn very slowly with negative pressure. Once the correct position is found, rest the hand holding the syringe against the patient's leg. The usual dose is 50 mg hydrocortisone acetate, 40 mg methylprednisolone, or 20 mg triamcinolone (hex) acetonide. If injecting steroid do not completely aspirate the joint, so as to permit free diffusion of steroid around the cavity.

Prepatella bursitis—Several bursae are present on the lower surface of the patella and patellar tendon. While bursitis will usually respond to using a kneeling pad, some cases are sufficiently painful to warrant injecting 25 mg hydrocortisone acetate into the most tender area.

Shoulder

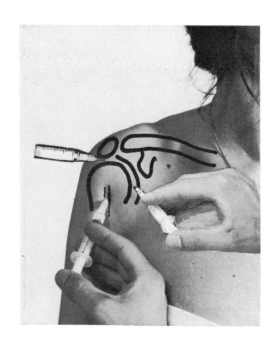

The shoulder joint is most easily entered anteriorly: this route is used for aspiration, frozen shoulder, and synovitis. With the patient seated and his arm relaxed against the side of the chest, feel for the space between the head of the humerus and the glenoid cap, about 1 cm below the coracoid process. If in doubt, rotate the humerus by moving the extended hand outwards and feel the head moving under the fingers. Insert the needle into the space with a slight medial angle. It should enter the joint easily, almost to the length of a green needle. The usual dose is 25-50 mg hydrocortisone acetate.

The lateral approach is used mainly for subacromial bursitis or the painful arc syndrome. Feel for the lateral tip of the acromium and insert the needle just below it in a medial direction with a slight downward slant until the tip reaches the humeral head. Gradually withdraw the needle with gentle pressure on the plunger: when the needle point is in the subacromial bursa a sudden drop in resistance will be felt. Injection will often reproduce the symptoms of the painful arc syndrome; if it does not, angle the needle in different directions until the pain is reproduced. Mixing local anaesthetic with the steroid is a useful diagnostic test, as the shoulder movements (or symptoms) should be improved after a few minutes. A second injection after a few days is often required.

Bicipital tendinitis is one cause of shoulder pain and is detected by finding tenderness over the tendon when the arm is externally rotated. Insert the needle almost parallel to the tendon—if it enters the tendon there will be resistance to the injection—then withdraw slightly and inject 25 mg hydrocortisone acetate into the tendon sheath and 25 mg direct into the shoulder joint, as part of the tendon is intra-articular.

Elbow

Care is needed to differentiate between the possible sites of pain. Tennis and golfer's elbow are the common reasons for injection. The elbow is not an easy joint to inject, except in the presence of an effusion. The lateral approach is just proximal to the radial head, with the elbow flexed at 90°. Palpate the radial head while rotating the patient's hand, and locate the proximal end. Insert the needle between this and the lateral epicondyle at about 90° to the skin. The posterior approach may be used, again with the elbow at 90°, with the needle aimed between the olecranon process and the lateral epicondyle.

Tennis elbow—Carefully locate the site of maximal pain over the annular ligament of the radius and muscle attachments to it or to the lateral humeral epicondyle. Using a green or blue needle, infiltrate (with considerable pressure) 25 mg hydrocortisone acetate and 1 ml local anaesthetic in and around the area of maximal tenderness, reinserting the needle down to bone in several areas without completely withdrawing it. After some five minutes check that the local tenderness has disappeared. A second injection is often needed after a few days.

Golfer's elbow—Once again, carefully localise the maximal point of tenderness at the insertion of muscles into the medial epicondyle of the humerus and medial ligament, and inject as for tennis elbow. Remember to palpate and avoid the ulnar nerve in the groove below the medial epicondyle.

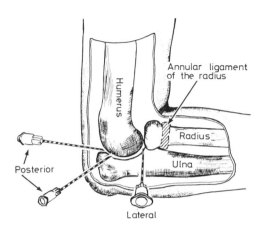

Wrist

The easiest site for injecting the wrist is just distal to the ulnar head, on the dorsal surface of the wrist and slightly inside (to the radial side). In theory several separate synovial cavities may exist, but in practice, particularly with persistent synovitis, usually all of these interconnect. Carefully palpate the space between the ulnar head and the lunate, and insert the needle at right angles to the skin between the extensor tendons to the ring and little fingers to a depth of about 1·0-1·5 cm. With careful palpation and marking the needle will slip into a space between bones. The usual dose is 25 mg hydrocortisone acetate.

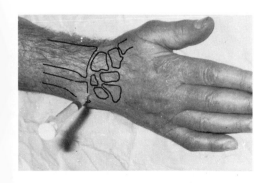

De Quervain's tenosynovitis—Tenosynovitis may occur in synovial sheaths surrounding the tendons of extensor pollicis longus and occasionally abductor pollicis longus as they pass through the extensor retinaculum on the dorsum of the wrist, and is usually apparent as a tender swelling along the tendons. Carefully palpate the swelling and insert the needle almost parallel to the skin, aiming it into the centre of the swelling. If the needle point is in the tendon injection will be difficult. Gradually withdraw the needle, with gentle pressure on the plunger, until free, easy flow occurs. The usual dose is 25 mg hydrocortisone acetate, but volume may be a problem: inject slowly, especially after 0·5 ml.

Aspiration and injection of joints

Hand

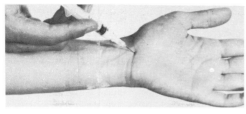

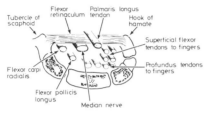

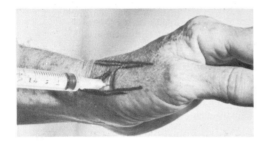

Carpal tunnel—On the palmar surface of the hand the carpal tunnel is bridged by the flexor retinaculum, which runs between the hook of the hamate and the crest of the trapezium. These bony points are easily palpated at the level of the distal transverse skin crease. Insert the needle at right angles to the skin at this level, preferably closer to the hamate on the ulnar side, to avoid the median nerve, which is close to the trapezium, and superficial veins. The usual dose is 25 mg hydrocortisone acetate.

Palmar flexor tendons—Tenosynovitis of the finger flexor tendon sheaths may present as pain and difficulty on flexing the finger or as trigger finger. In the former case the tendon sheath feels thickened; in trigger finger a nodule on the tendon may be felt "popping" as the finger is flexed and extended. Carefully palpate the tendon in the palm with the fingers extended; insert the needle at the proximal skin crease of the finger, almost parallel to the course of the tendon and pointing towards the palm. Then proceed as for De Quervain's tenosynovitis.

First carpometacarpal joint of thumb—Palpate the proximal margin of the first metacarpal bone in the anatomical snuffbox: flexion of the thumb into the palm of the hand will widen the joint space. Select a site between the long extensor and long abductor muscles; locate and avoid the radial artery. Insert the needle, pointing it at the base of the little finger, to a depth of about 1 cm. The usual dose is 25 mg hydrocortisone acetate.

Percutaneous synovial biopsy of knee

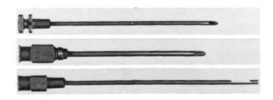

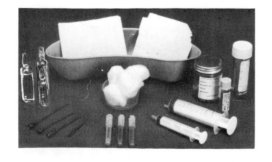

Synovial biopsy is much simpler than open biopsy and usually yields equivalent information. Use of the Parker-Pearson biopsy needle has been described in other joints but in practice is confined to the knee. The following instruments are required on the trolley: a Parker-Pearson needle, small scalpel blade, saline, local anaesthetic, choice of needles and syringes, sterile pack, and gloves.

Generously infiltrate with local anaesthetic an area medial to the upper half of the patella down to the synovial membrane. If synovial fluid is required for diagnostic purposes withdraw it at this stage and replace it with 20 ml of saline. If the joint is not well distended with fluid simulate an effusion with 20 ml saline.

Incise the skin with the small scalpel needle and insert the cannula and trocar through the incision and through muscle into the joint. Reassure the patient that he may feel pressure but not pain, and infiltrate with more local anaesthetic if necessary. The cannula and trocar can usually be felt passing through the synovium, and synovial fluid will run from the cannula as the trocar is withdrawn. Angle the trocar into the suprapatellar pouch and insert the biopsy needle, so that the specimen is from the synovium under the quadriceps muscle. It is helpful to press the synovium down on to the needle with the heel of the hand and to move the cannula and needle to excise tissue rather than pull it off. The needle is then withdrawn, and synovium may be lifted out with a hypodermic needle. If the cannula is left in several specimens may be obtained.

BONE-MARROW ASPIRATION AND TREPHINE BIOPSY

S KNOWLES   A V HOFFBRAND

Indications

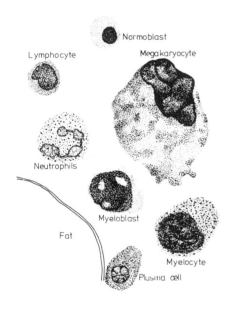

Bone-marrow examination is essential in the investigation of many haematological disorders. It may provide a diagnosis suspected from the clinical features and peripheral blood examination or occasionally gives a previously unsuspected diagnosis. It is also useful in certain diseases for assessing the extent or response to treatment. Bone-marrow fragments may be aspirated and spread on slides, as for a blood film, or a core of bone and marrow may be obtained intact and histologically sectioned (trephine biopsy). The table shows the main indications for one or both of these tests. In general, aspiration is used to show the morphology of individual haemopoietic cells and to obtain material for ancillary tests, whereas a trephine gives a more representative view of the cellularity of the marrow and allows infiltrations to be recognised.

The investigations are limited by the small size of the samples and consequent sampling errors. Infiltrations may be missed, and the cellularity may vary from site to site. Nevertheless, the tests provide a considerable amount of information and should always be considered before a large battery of investigations is requested, particularly if these investigations are time consuming and costly and may prove to have been irrelevant once the marrow appearances are known.

Indications for bone-marrow aspiration and trephine biopsy

Indications	Ancillary tests
Bone-marrow aspiration*	
Unexplained anaemia (particularly when reticulocyte count low)	
Macrocytic anaemia (to distinguish megaloblastic from normoblastic erythropoiesis)	Deoxyuridine suppression test
Granulocytopenia or thrombocytopenia, or both (to distinguish failure of production from peripheral consumption)	
Suspected acute leukaemia (and to monitor treatment) and myelodysplastic syndromes	Cytochemistry, cytogenetics, electron microscopy, cell surface markers, enzyme assays, semi-solid agar culture
Suspected myeloma	Immunofluorescence
Suspected lipidoses	
Diagnosis of certain infections—for example, tuberculosis, kala-azar	Appropriate microbiological culture
Bone-marrow aspiration and trephine†	
Pancytopenia—for example, aplastic anaemia, hypersplenism	
Chronic leukaemia	Cytogenetics (in chronic granulocytic leukaemia)
Myeloproliferative diseases—for example, polycythaemia, thrombocythaemia, myelosclerosis	Cytogenetics
Suspected infiltration by, for example, lymphoma, carcinoma, granuloma	Immunofluorescence or immunoperoxidase studies in non-Hodgkin's lymphoma
If repeated "dry taps" on attempted aspiration, perform trephine biopsy	

*Routine stains are Romanowsky (for example, May-Grünwald Giemsa) and iron; results available in one to two hours.
†Routine stains for the trephine biopsy are haematoxylin and eosin, and reticulin; results available in seven days (unless rapid decalcification used).

Bone-marrow aspiration and trephine biopsy

Needles

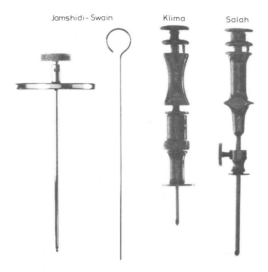

Jamshidi-Swain   Klima   Salah

Aspiration needles (the Salah or Klima) are short and stout and should have a sharpened bevel, a well-fitting and easily removable stylet, and an adjustable guard for use in sternal aspirations. For a trephine biopsy the Jamshidi-Swain needle is favoured. This has a radially tapered distal cutting tip, which prevents the specimen from being crushed or plugged in the needle.

Sites

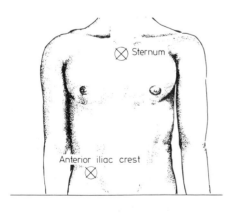

Sternum

Anterior iliac crest

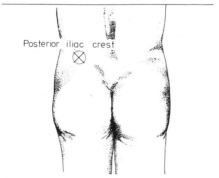

Posterior iliac crest

Aspiration may be done at the following sites.

Sternum—At the level of the second or third interspace, just to one side of the midline, with the patient in a semi-recumbent or supine position. This site should be used only for patients over 12 years old. It is the easiest site from which to obtain the most cellular marrow but causes the greatest patient apprehension.

Posterior iliac crest—May be used for any patient over 1 year old. The patient is placed in the right or left lateral position with the back comfortably flexed, and the uppermost crest is used. This site can be a difficult landmark to find in an obese patient, but several attempts to obtain marrow can be made in the same area.

Anterior iliac crest—May be used in adults with the patient supine. A site is chosen 2·5-5 cm posterior to the anterior superior iliac spine and beneath the palpable lip.

Tibia—For use in children less than 1 year old. The flat triangular area at the proximal end of the medial surface of the tibia, just below the tibial tubercle, is chosen.

Trephine biopsy should be undertaken only at the posterior iliac crest, and, since both an aspirate and a trephine biopsy specimen are often necessary, this site is commonly used. Biopsy specimens may, however, be taken from other sites—for example, where an x-ray film or bone scan suggests a definite lesion.

Technique for aspiration

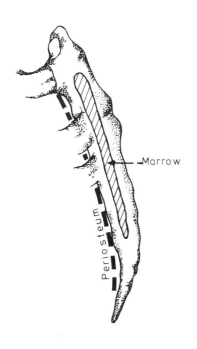

Sedation is not usually needed except for children and apprehensive adults. A clean, no-touch technique should be used, but in patients with neutropenia a mask and gloves are recommended. The patient is positioned appropriately for the site chosen and the area cleaned with chlorhexidine or iodine and surrounded with sterile towels. The bony landmarks are identified and the overlying skin and periosteum infiltrated with up to 5 ml of 2% plain lignocaine. Check that the needle is sharp, the stylet easily removable, and the guard mobile. (For iliac crest and tibial procedures the guard may be removed.) With one hand identifying the landmarks and keeping the overlying tissues taut, push the needle through the skin and subcutaneous tissues. For sternal aspiration the guard should be adjusted when the periosteum is reached, so that only a further 5 mm advancement is possible. The needle is held at right angles to the bone and with firm pressure and a clockwise-counterclockwise action pushed through the outer cortex until a sensation of decreased resistance is felt when the marrow cavity is entered. The stylet is removed, a 10 or 20 ml syringe attached to the needle, and with gentle suction up to 0·5 ml of marrow aspirated into the syringe for morphological examination. Any greater volume will result in increasing contamination with peripheral blood. A second volume may be aspirated into another syringe for ancillary studies.

If no marrow is aspirated the needle is rotated or the stylet replaced and the needle cautiously advanced or retracted. If marrow is still unobtainable, a different site together with a clean needle should be used and possibly a trephine specimen taken.

Preparation of bone-marrow slides

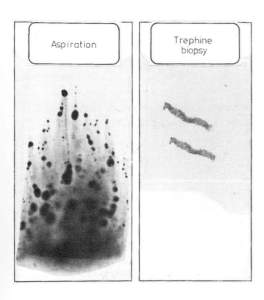

Smears must be made promptly before the specimen clots. It is a technique that requires practice, and badly made films render the aspirate uninterpretable. An accompanying technician may be needed to make the films or, if necessary, the sample may be placed into disodium EDTA for a few minutes until the laboratory is reached. A paediatric tube should be used to avoid an excess of anticoagulant.

When marrow films are prepared a drop of the aspirate is placed 1 cm from the end of a clean slide. Excess blood is aspirated with a Pasteur pipette or a second needle and syringe leaving marrow particles behind. Some workers concentrate all the particles on a separate slide or watch glass. By using a second smooth slide or spreader, a 3-5 cm film is made from the particles in the same manner as for peripheral blood. The particles should leave a trail of cells. At least eight slides should be available for staining. Romanowsky (for example, May-Grünwald Giemsa) and iron stains are performed routinely, and cytochemical examination of other slides may be needed. Additional material should be put in the appropriate medium with an anticoagulant for special tests—for example, cytogenetic and biochemical studies, etc—or into a microbiological culture medium.

Bone-marrow aspiration and trephine biopsy

Jamshidi-Swain trephine

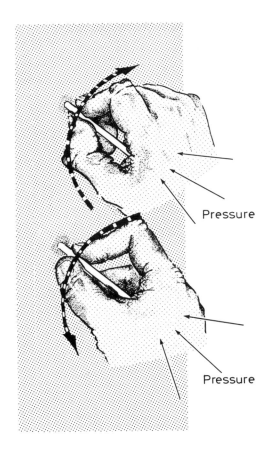

Pressure

Pressure

The patient is positioned and prepared as for posterior crest aspiration. The skin overlying the crest is incised with a scalpel blade, or the site of entry of a previous aspiration is used. With the handle of the needle grasped in the palm of the hand and the stylet locked in position the needle is pushed through the subcutaneous tissues until it reaches the posterior crest. It is then slowly advanced with firm pressure in an alternating clockwise-counterclockwise motion in the direction of the anterior superior iliac spine until a sensation of decreased resistance is felt. The stylet is removed and the needle further advanced until 2-3 cm of marrow is obtained. The needle is then withdrawn 2-3 mm and with less pressure advanced 2-3 mm further in a different direction, which breaks the specimen at the distal cutting edge of the needle. The instrument containing the biopsy sample is then withdrawn by rotation along its axis with quick full twists.

The specimen is removed from the needle by introducing the probe through the distal cutting end. The biopsy can be dabbed on to or rolled across a slide before being placed into fixative for routine staining. After decalcification sections are stained routinely with haematoxylin and eosin and for reticulin.

Risks and aftercare

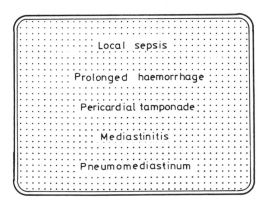

Local sepsis

Prolonged haemorrhage

Pericardial tamponade

Mediastinitis

Pneumomediastinum

In severe coagulation disorders (for example, haemophilia, severe disseminated intravascular coagulation) the procedure should be undertaken only when the defect has been corrected by appropriate plasma fraction replacements. A trephine biopsy in such conditions might give rise to prolonged haemorrhage. Thrombocytopenia alone does not usually present a major problem.

Failure to use the guard when performing sternal aspiration could give rise to complete penetration of the bone with a resultant fatal haemorrhage, pericardial tamponade, mediastinitis, or pneumomediastinum. Local sepsis is extremely rare except in patients with severe neutropenia, for whom sterile precautions should be taken.

After the procedure a plaster is applied, and firm pressure over the site for a few minutes is recommended (for longer if the patient has a haemostatic defect).

SUPRAPUBIC CATHETERISATION

P HILTON   S L STANTON

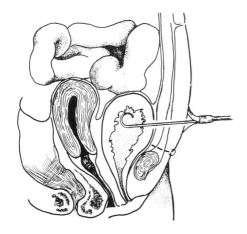

Suprapubic catheterisation is the technique of draining the bladder by a catheter passed through the anterior abdominal wall. It may be performed as an open or closed procedure, and either method may be carried out in the ward under local anaesthesia or in the theatre under general anaesthesia. Although most of the following comments relate to closed catheterisation in women, using the Bonanno catheter, the same general principles of insertion and subsequent management apply in all cases.

Indications

Pelvic surgery

Acute retention of urine

Urethral trauma
and surgery

Management after pelvic surgery—All gynaecological, urological, and rectal operations may be associated with postoperative urinary retention. The advantage of a suprapubic catheter is that the patient's ability to void can be assessed without removing the catheter. This appreciably reduces patient discomfort, nursing time, and urinary infection, since repeated catheterisations become unnecessary.

Acute retention of urine—In men with acute urinary retention the passage of a urethral catheter is often painful and, if the first attempt is unsuccessful, repeated attempts may lead to the formation of a false passage, infection, and stricture. In women these problems are uncommon, but nevertheless retention is often treated by repeated urethral catheterisation when one suprapubic catheterisation would suffice.

Urethral trauma, urethral or bladder-neck surgery, and repair of vesical or urethral fistula—In these conditions urethral catheterisation may not only further damage the mucosa but also encourage local oedema and delay healing.

Contraindications

Inability to distend bladder

Carcinoma of bladder

Gross haematuria

Recent cystotomy

Inability to distend the bladder—Ideally the bladder should be distended with 500 ml, though with experience 300 ml may be adequate. At lower volumes the danger of perforating the bowel becomes too great to justify the closed procedure.

Known or suspected carcinoma of the bladder—The risk of implanting malignant cells in the fistulous track makes even suspected carcinoma an absolute contraindication.

Gross haematuria or clot retention—The catheters used for closed cystostomy are generally of fine calibre and should not be used when there is a risk of occlusion by clot. A larger catheter (22 French gauge) inserted by open cystotomy is more suitable.

Recent cystotomy—An open technique at the time of operation is preferable to closed catheterisation, as this may disrupt the vesical suture line.

Suprapubic catheterisation

Types of catheter

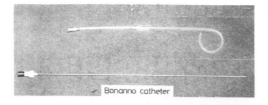

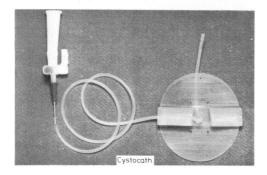

Bonanno catheter

Cystocath

Bonanno (6 French gauge)—Two small tabs secured by sutures permit insertion close to a suprapubic transverse incision. The catheter may be left in place for around three weeks and is ideal for postoperative use.

Cystocath (8 French gauge)—A large adhesive flange permits secure attachment for long-term drainage. This catheter is less suitable when there is a recent abdominal incision.

Argyle Ingram trocar catheter (12 and 16 French gauge) is more solid in construction than other designs but uncomfortable for a mobile patient. It is secured by an intravesical balloon with a flange sutured to the skin; an irrigation channel is provided.

Stamey percutaneous catheter (10 French gauge) is secured by Malecot-type flanges and is not tethered to the skin.

Foley catheters may also be inserted suprapubically.

MANUFACTURERS—Bonanno catheter: Becton-Dickinson and Co; Cystocath: Dow-Corning Corporation; Argyle Ingram trocar catheter: Sherwood Medical Inc; Stamey percutaneous catheter: Vance Products Inc.

Procedure

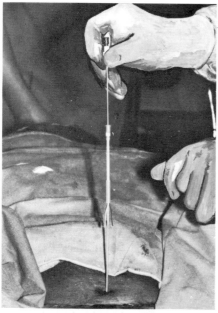

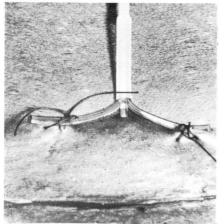

For immediate postoperative bladder drainage the catheter is inserted under general or regional anaesthesia; otherwise local infiltration is perfectly satisfactory.

The following equipment should be assembled beforehand: 1 in 100 aqueous Savlon, for urethral preparation; 1 in 30 alcoholic Savlon, for skin preparation; swabs or cotton-wool balls; a disposable urethral catheter—for example, Nelaton, 12-14 French gauge; intravenous infusion set with 500 ml saline; local anaesthetic—for example, 5-10 ml of 1-2% lignocaine; syringe and needles; No 11 scalpel blade; catheter pack; 00 silk suture; urine drainage bag; and tape—for example, Sleek.

Whatever the type of catheter used, the manufacturer's instructions should be studied beforehand by the operator and nursing staff.

When the catheter is to be used postoperatively the bladder must first be filled. Using standard aseptic techniques, a urethral catheter is passed and 400-500 ml sterile saline instilled via the infusion set. The suprapubic area should be prepared, the point of insertion being in the midline 3 cm above the symphysis pubis. In obese patients the catheter is most easily inserted in the suprapubic crease. When local anaesthesia is used the point of insertion should be infiltrated down to the bladder with 1-2% lignocaine. A small stab incision with a No 11 scalpel blade facilitates catheter introduction. The catheter, assembled according to the manufacturer's instructions, is introduced through the incision with a firm thrust in a slightly caudal direction. Resistance should be minimal once the bladder is entered, but correct siting is confirmed by free flow of urine when the stylet or trocar is disengaged.

The catheter may be advanced until its flange is flat against the skin, while at the same time the needle is withdrawn. The catheter is fixed to the skin by a suture, adhesive, tape, or balloon inflation as appropriate. It is connected to a drainage bag, which should also be secured to the skin to prevent dragging. The bladder is drained and the urethral catheter removed.

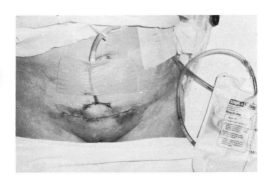

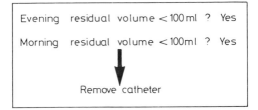

Evening residual volume < 100 ml ? Yes

Morning residual volume < 100 ml ? Yes

Remove catheter

Subsequent management—The catheter should be left on continuous drainage until the patient is to attempt voiding (day 2 postoperatively). The adaptor or drainage connection (not the catheter itself) is then clamped and the patient encouraged to void normally. If she is unable to void or becomes distressed the clamp should be released. If she achieves normal voiding the residual volume should be checked after eight hours. The residual volume is obtained by emptying the drainage bag, allowing the patient to void, and then unclamping the catheter for five to 15 minutes, depending on its calibre.

Our usual practice is to leave the catheter on continuous drainage overnight until the evening residual volume is less than 100 ml. The catheter is then clamped overnight, and if the patient has successfully voided during the night and the residual volume is less than 100 ml the catheter is removed.

If prophylactic chemotherapy is not used during catheterisation we recommend that urine samples should be obtained every three days for culture and sensitivity tests.

Complications

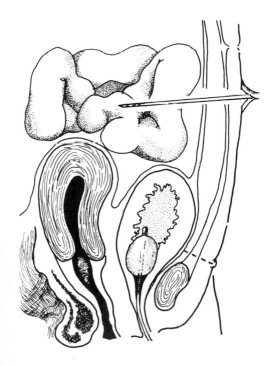

Failure to enter the bladder is rarely a problem if the bladder is adequately distended beforehand. If free flow of urine is not observed when the catheter and stylet are disengaged the catheter should be aspirated with a syringe. If urine is not obtained the whole catheter should be removed and resited after further distension of the bladder.

Bowel injury—If contents of the small or large bowel are aspirated into the syringe the catheter should be removed and resited. Antibiotic treatment should be started: we recommend a combination of metronidazole and a cephalosporin. Close observation of pulse and blood pressure should be maintained postoperatively. If this complication arises during insertion of a rigid catheter of larger bore (12-16 French gauge) we would recommend more active treatment: laparotomy should be undertaken, and if the catheter is left in place this may permit more easy localisation of the site of perforation.

Detachment of the catheter from the skin can usually be managed by resuturing or retaping.

Leakage around the catheter appears to be less of a problem with suprapubic than with urethral catheters. It can usually be controlled with antispasmodic treatment, using emepronium bromide, flavoxate hydrochloride, or propantheline bromide.

Fracture of the catheter or incomplete removal—Particularly with fine catheters bearing multiple side holes there is a small risk of fracture during removal. A senior nurse should always check the catheter to ensure that it is complete. When doubt exists radiological confirmation and, if necessary, cystoscopic retrieval should be performed.

Haematuria may occur on the first day after insertion due to trauma caused by the catheterisation, or later due to cystitis or to irritation of bladder mucosa by the catheter. A catheter specimen of urine should be cultured, but in the absence of infection haematuria will usually settle spontaneously.

LUMBAR PUNCTURE

C CLOUGH   J M S PEARCE

Indications for performing lumbar puncture

Diagnostic tests

Introducing contrast media

Introducing chemotherapy

Lumbar puncture should not be indulged in idly as a result of diagnostic bankruptcy nor in place of a neurological opinion. Though it may be informative in certain patients with coma or stroke it should not be done blindly as an immediate procedure until other diagnostic tests have been performed.

There are three main indications: (a) for diagnostic purposes (see table); (b) for introducing contrast media; and (c) for introducing chemotherapeutic agents—for example, in meningitis or leukaemia.

Indications for performing lumbar puncture for diagnosis	Tests
Suspected subarachnoid haemorrhage	Blood, xanthochromia
Selected strokes, but not routinely	Red blood cells, protein
Myelopathies and suspected multiple sclerosis (but not for suspected cord compression)	Protein, IgG, or gammaglobulin
Peripheral neuropathies—for example, Guillain-Barré syndrome	Cells, protein
Infections of central nervous system (bacterial meningitis; tuberculosis; acute and subacute encephalitides; neurosyphilis; viral, fungal, and protozoal meningitis)	Cells, protein, treponemal haemagglutinating antibody (or other specific tests), glucose, culture, virology, special stains and antibodies

Contraindications

Raised intracranial pressure

Suspected cord compression

Local sepsis

The contraindications to lumbar puncture must be kept in mind whenever the procedure is being considered. These are: (1) Raised intracranial pressure—papilloedema or a history suggesting raised intracranial pressure (even in the absence of signs) should lead to a neurological consultation and a computerised axial tomography scan or angiogram. To proceed with the puncture in the absence of these investigations could lead to fatal "coning." (2) Suspected cord compression—in many isolated spinal cord lesions it is impossible to distinguish an intrinsic lesion (for example, multiple sclerosis) from extrinsic compression. Myelography with simultaneous cerebrospinal fluid examination is then necessary, rather than a separate lumbar puncture. (3) Local sepsis—meningitis is a rare complication of lumbar puncture, but puncture should not be performed if there is skin sepsis.

Procedure

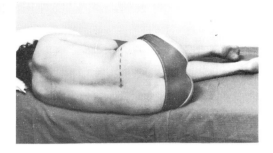

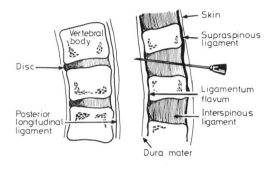

The most important factor in achieving an easy lumbar puncture is the correct positioning of the patient. The procedure should be explained to the patient and he should be comfortable and relaxed.

Place the patient on his left side with his back right up against the edge of the bed or firm trolley. Both legs are flexed towards the chest: place a pillow between the legs to ensure that the back is vertical. The neck should be slightly flexed.

Masks and gloves should be worn. Clean the skin with iodine (or other antiseptic) and spirit and then position sterile drapes. Use a gauge 18 lumbar puncture needle, and check that the stylet is flush with the end and that the manometer is intact and fits the needle hub. A 22- to 25-gauge needle is preferable in younger patients without osteophytes and in thin patients.

Palpate the anterior-superior iliac spine. The interspace perpendicularly beneath it is that at L3-4. Since the spinal cord ends at L1-2 the spaces above and below L3-4 are equally acceptable sites. Palpate the spinous processes superior to the chosen interspace: the needle will be inserted about 1 cm inferior to the tip of the process.

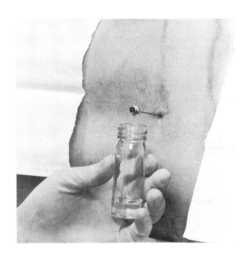

Draw up 5 ml of lignocaine 2% plain and, stretching the skin evenly over the interspace, infiltrate the skin and deeper tissues.

Allow at least one minute for the lignocaine to work then introduce the needle. Make sure that the needle is 90° to the back, with its bevel in the sagittal plane and pointing slightly to the head. Push the needle through the resistance of the superficial supraspinous ligament. The interspinous ligament is then easily negotiated. At about 4-7 cm the firmer resistance of the ligamentum flavum is felt, when an extra push will result in a popping sensation as the dura is breached.

The needle should now lie in the subarachnoid space, and when the stylet is withdrawn clear colourless fluid should drip out.

Dry tap: usually failure of technique

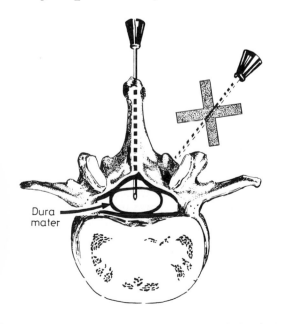

If no fluid emerges or it does not flow easily rotate the needle, because a flap of dura may be lying against the bevel. If there is still no fluid reinsert the stylet and cautiously advance, withdrawing the stylet after each movement. Pain radiating down either leg indicates that the needle is too lateral and has hit nerve roots. Withdraw the needle almost completely, check the patient's position, and reinsert in the midline.

If the needle meets total obstruction do not force it as the needle may be lying against an intervertebral disc and could damage it. Again, withdraw the needle, check its position, and reinsert. If there is complete failure move one space up or down depending on the original position. The procedure may be easier if the patient is sitting up.

A dry tap is usually due to a failure of technique. After two or three attempts a colleague should be invited to show his superior skill. Rare causes of a genuine dry tap are arachnoiditis and infiltrations of the meninges.

Lumbar puncture

Manometry

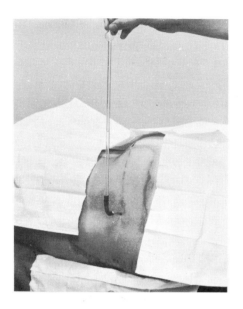

Once free flow of CSF is established the pressure should be measured. The manometer is connected to the end of the needle directly or via a two-way tap. An assistant holds the top end, and the resting pressure is recorded (normal 80-180 mm H_2O CSF). Queckenstedt's test is performed by asking the assistant to compress the jugular vein, which should cause a quick rise of at least 40 mm, which should be recorded. The test should never be used in place of myelography to show a spinal tumour or disc lesion. Its use is now confined to hospitals without neuroradiological facilities.

Spinal block causes a failure of free rise and fall (positive Queckenstedt) and is usually accompanied by yellowish CSF with a high protein content (Froin's syndrome).

The commonest cause of low CSF pressure is bad needle placement, but if the low pressure is genuine no attempt should be made to aspirate as the cause may be obstruction of CSF flow caused by cerebellar tonsil herniation or spinal block. In either case a neurological opinion is needed.

A slightly raised CSF pressure in a very anxious or fat patient may be ignored. Pressures over 250 mm are abnormal and should be investigated. If a greatly raised pressure is discovered in a clear fluid the CSF should be collected from the manometer and the needle withdrawn. The patient should be nursed flat and a neurologist or neurosurgeon consulted.

Specimens for diagnosis

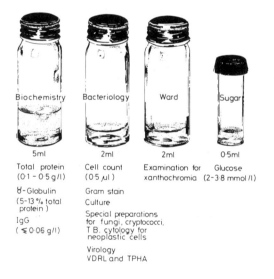

Biochemistry	Bacteriology	Ward	Sugar
5ml	2ml	2ml	0·5ml
Total protein (0·1 - 0·5 g/l)	Cell count (0·5 µl)	Examination for xanthochromia	Glucose (2-3·8 mmol/l)
४-Globulin (5-13% total protein)	Gram stain		
IgG (≤0·06 g/l)	Culture		
	Special preparations for fungi, cryptococci, T.B. cytology for neoplastic cells		
	Virology VDRL and TPHA		

Eight to 10 ml of CSF is usually collected, depending on the particular investigation. The normal *basic* requirements are: pressure, cells, and total protein. There are no routine tests, and additional investigations should be requested as necessary with the guidance of the local laboratory. Lange curves and chloride estimations rarely give useful information.

A ward specimen is useful in suspected subarachnoid haemorrhage, where xanthochromia (a yellow discoloration) in the supernatant can be seen. It is also a useful spare for "mislaid specimens."

Even the most careful lumbar puncture can be bedevilled by bloodstaining. Bloody fluid should be collected in three tubes. A traumatic tap can be distinguished from subarachnoid haemorrhage in three ways.

Firstly, blood due to trauma forms streams in an otherwise clear CSF, while the CSF of subarachnoid bleeding is diffusely bloodstained.

Secondly, on centrifugation or standing the supernatant is colourless in a traumatic tap but xanthochromic in subarachnoid haemorrhage. The only exception is that a clear supernatant may rarely occur if the lumbar puncture is done within six hours of a subarachnoid haemorrhage occurring.

Thirdly, the first three consecutive specimens of CSF in a traumatic tap show clearing of the blood and usually become colourless, with a corresponding fall of the red cell count.

Aftercare and complications

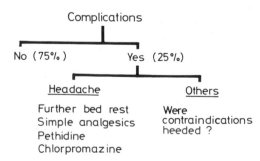

Once the specimens have been collected the needle should be removed, a plaster applied, and the patient nursed flat for an arbitrary 24 hours. Some experienced operators prefer to nurse the patient prone, slightly head down, for as long as can be tolerated after the procedure. This may mechanically aid closure of the hole in the dura. Three-quarters of patients have no symptoms. Headache occurs for 24-48 hours in the remainder but is severe in only half. Headache should be treated with further rest horizontally in bed, with simple analgesics, but with pethidine and chlorpromazine if necessary. If the contraindications are heeded there should be no other complications.

PASSING A NASOGASTRIC TUBE

JENNIFER LEWIS   A TUCKER

Indications

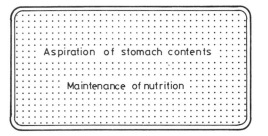

Aspiration of stomach contents

Maintenance of nutrition

There are two main indications for passing a nasogastric tube. One is to aspirate stomach contents, either as a diagnostic test—for example, using pentagastrin—or as a therapeutic measure—for example, in the "acute abdomen." The other is to maintain nutrition of the patient, either when he should not swallow—for example, after pharyngeal surgery—or when he cannot swallow—for example, in postcricoid carcinoma, before treatment.

Equipment

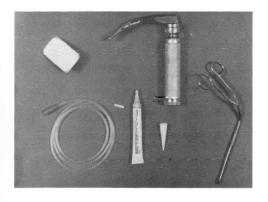

Nasogastric tube—Select a large (say, 16 French gauge) rather than a small tube, as this will be less likely to block during use or form a false passage during its introduction. If the tube is to be used only for feeding a fine-bore (1 mm) tube with a wire introducer may be chosen, particularly for use with proprietary feeding preparations.

Lubricating jelly—Although a simple water-soluble jelly (for example, K-Y) is usually used, lignocaine gel 2% antiseptic may be more comfortable for the patient, especially if the tube does not pass at the first attempt.

Syringe (60 ml) for aspirating.

Blue litmus paper to test the aspirated fluid for acid and confirm that the tip of the tube is in the stomach.

Procedure

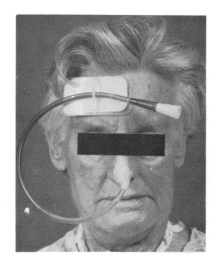

A sterile technique is not required, although simple hygiene should be observed. Explain the procedure to the patient. Lubricate the nose with lignocaine jelly via the supplied applicator, and allow this to take effect. Gravity will assist the passage of the fluid to the back of the nose.

With the patient sitting, introduce the lubricated tube along the floor of the nose. Resistance will be felt as the tip reaches the nasopharynx, which is the least comfortable part of the procedure. Ask him to swallow (helped by water from a spouted feeding beaker if not contraindicated), while continuing to advance the tube, which should pass down the oesophagus without resistance. At 40 cm the gastro-oesophageal junction is reached. Pass this and anchor the tube to the nose with adhesive tape.

Passing a nasogastric tube

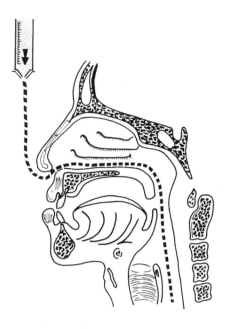

Test the aspirate for acid. If there is no aspirate to test, connect to the tube a 60 ml syringe filled with air and auscultate the stomach while an assistant slowly empties the syringe. It is important that the operator should not leave the patient until the position of the tip is confirmed, and if in doubt an *x*-ray film should be obtained—most tubes have a radio-opaque tip, and fine PVC tubes are themselves radio-opaque.

If the tube is to be used for feeding purposes the first feed should consist of water.

Problems

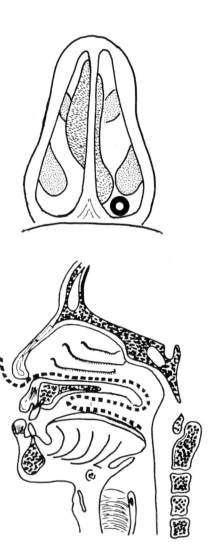

Choking usually indicates that the tube has entered the trachea and should be withdrawn immediately.

Difficulties in passing the tube may occur at any point along the route:

Nose—Pass the tube along the floor of the nose and not towards the bridge. If one nostril is narrowed by a deviation of the nasal septum, use the other side, although there is often a "tunnel" along the floor of the nose which can be used. In the event of persistent difficulty select a smaller tube and consider using a topical vasoconstrictor (for example, ephedrine 0·5% drops).

Oropharynx—Reflex gagging by the patient may direct the tube into the mouth. There are various ways of dealing with this problem: try the following in order. (*a*) Repeated attempts. Withdraw the tip into the nasopharynx and advance again until it passes into the oesophagus. (*b*) Cool the tube in a refrigerator or ice to stiffen it so that it is less likely to coil. (*c*) Observe the passage of the tube through the mouth with a depressor on the tongue. Use a pair of long forceps (for example, McGill's) to guide the tube down. (*d*) As a final measure, give the patient a benzocaine lozenge 10 mg to suck for 10 minutes. Then lay him flat, remove the head of the bed, and use a Mackintosh laryngoscope to visualise the oropharynx. Direct the tube past the base of the tongue as an assistant introduces it through the nose. There is no need to visualise the larynx, for as long as the tube passes along the posterior pharyngeal wall it should enter the oesophagus.

Oesophagus—A stricture or pharyngeal pouch may prevent the tube from passing, and this is probably the only indication for a general anaesthetic.

Tubes may be left in place for long periods, but strapping is best changed daily.

Obstruction of the tube may be due to blockage by its contents or to the tube twisting on itself. A blockage should be cleared by flushing (citrate solution seems to help), and a twisted tube corrected by partially withdrawing it until it functions again, then relocating it and confirming its position. Fine-bore tubes have a greater tendency to be regurgitated.

Perforation of the oesophagus is extremely unlikely in the absence of oesophageal disease.

TAKING BLOOD AND PUTTING UP A DRIP IN YOUNG CHILDREN

ANDREW WHITELAW   BERNARD VALMAN

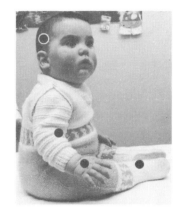

Blood may be obtained from young children by heel prick or thumb prick, but venepuncture is essential for blood culture, coagulation studies, and tests requiring more than 1 ml of blood. Suitable superficial veins include the antecubital veins and those on the back of the wrist, the foot, and the scalp. Using the external jugular vein is frightening for children. The internal jugular and femoral veins are potentially dangerous sites for venepuncture, as damage to adjacent structures may occur.

Capillary blood sampling

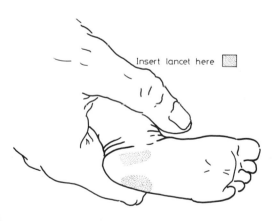

Insert lancet here

In babies under 6 months of age the heel is the ideal site for capillary blood sampling, but in older infants the thumb is better. The heel must be warm: if it is cold dip the foot into hand-warm water (40°C) for five minutes and then dry it thoroughly. Hold the foot by encircling the ball of the heel with your thumb and forefinger. Select a site on the side of the heel, wipe it with isopropyl alcohol, and allow it to dry. Do not use the ball or the back of the heel because a painful ulcer may form. Insert a disposable lancet about 2 mm and withdraw, cutting very slightly sideways. Wipe away the initial drop of blood with a dry cotton swab and then let the drops form and fall into the container. Squeeze and release your fingers around the calf to milk blood into the heel. Maintain the heel below the rest of the lower leg. Agitate the container to mix the blood with anticoagulant. When the required volume has been obtained wipe the heel and press with a clean cotton-wool ball. Apply a small plaster such as a Band-Aid.

Venepuncture

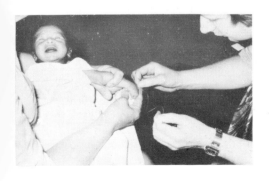

During venepuncture a nurse should hold and comfort the child. The arms should be examined under a good light. With manual compression round the upper arm the antecubital veins should be visible and palpable. With compression of the forearm and pronation and flexion of the wrist, veins should be visible and palpable on the back of the wrist. The antecubital veins are ideal because they are usually a good size and are unlikely to be needed for later infusions because there is movement at the elbow. Sterilise the skin with an alcohol swab and allow to dry. Use povidone-iodine if the blood is to be cultured.

Taking blood and putting up a drip in young children

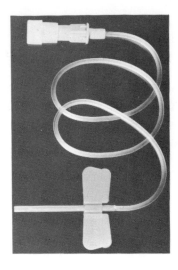

A 23-gauge butterfly needle is suitable for venepuncture because it is large enough to provide good blood flow but thin enough for small veins. A Y junction or an accessible straight vein is the best site to enter a vein. Insert the butterfly needle 0·5 cm distal to the planned point of entry into the vein. Advance the needle under the skin until it is at the junction or on top of the vein and then insert the needle into the vein, making sure that the skin is stretched distally to stretch the vein and prevent it from sliding away from the needle. Blood should flow into the tubing. Tape the butterfly needle in place with one strip of Micropore 1·3 cm ($\frac{1}{2}$ in) tape. Take the cap off the distal end of the butterfly-needle tube and connect a syringe. Be very patient when applying suction on the syringe, as overenthusiastic suction may stop blood flow altogether by pulling endothelium on to the end of the needle. With the butterfly needle taped to the skin, the syringe may be manipulated and changed without fear of dislodging the needle.

When the required volume has been withdrawn remove the tape, apply a cotton-wool or gauze swab to the vein, and gently withdraw the needle.

Putting up a drip

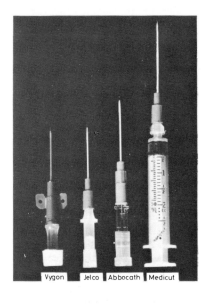

Vygon   Jelco   Abbocath   Medicut

Intravenous infusions are commonly needed in young children and infants for rehydration, drug treatment, inability to tolerate feeding, and surgery. For infants under 1 year, and particularly the newborn, scalp veins are a reliable site for infusions. Sites for older children include the back of the wrist, the forearm, and the ankle.

Butterfly needles are commonly used in infants because they are easy to insert and immobilise, particularly on the scalp. They are not ideal for older infants and toddlers because they are apt to cut out of the vein after a short time. The alternative is to use a plastic cannula such as the Medicut, Abbocath, Jelco Teflon Catheter Placement Unit, or Vygon Intraflon. These are preferable for limb veins because they do not cut out of the vein even when there is some movement.

Insertion of intravenous cannula

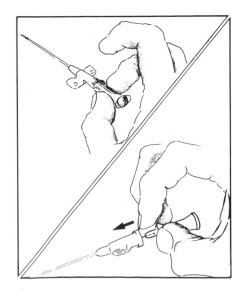

For insertion of an intravenous cannula a nurse holds the child and a rubber tourniquet is applied proximal to the selected limb vein. Assemble a paediatric giving set with a burette, a suitable intravenous fluid, and an intravenous infusion pump. Sterilise the skin over the vein with an alcohol swab and allow it to dry. Make a puncture in the skin distal to the vein with a No 1 (21 gauge) needle, then insert a 22-gauge needle catheter through the puncture. The previous skin puncture permits easier manipulation of the needle catheter under the skin. Insert the needle catheter into the vein. When blood flows back hold the shaft of the needle with the thumb and middle finger and advance the cannula with the forefinger. Alternatively, with your assistant holding the limb, hold the shaft of the needle still with the left hand and rotate the catheter, easing it forward over the end of the needle and into the vein for about 1 cm. Withdraw the needle. Gently rotate the catheter and insert it further if the vein will allow. Check that blood flows out of the catheter. Connect the giving set, take off the tourniquet, and check that the drip flows with gravity without subcutaneous swelling.

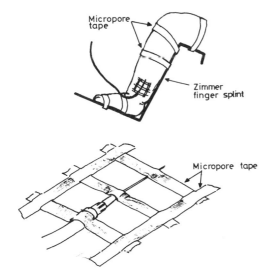

Fixation and immobilisation—There are many efficient ways of fixing an intravenous cannula. A square of gauze is placed over the point of insertion into the skin and secured by tape. A loop of the giving line should be taped to the side of the limb. To immobilise the wrist or ankle of an infant a wooden splint may be taped to the limb. A vigorous child may pull the catheter out, and the whole limb should be covered by a crêpe bandage or tube gauze. The limb of a newborn infant may be splinted by using two wooden tongue depressors, but we have recently been impressed by the use of metal finger splints (Zimmer), which may be bent to the angle of the knee, ankle, or wrist and retain their shape.

Scalp-vein infusion with butterfly needle

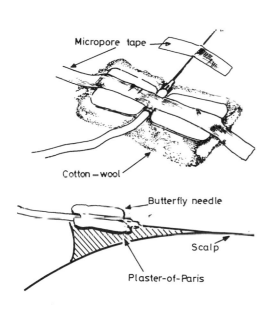

Explain to the mother that the needle is not going inside the skull, the procedure is painless after insertion, and the hair will grow back. If necessary, shave the hair on the temporoparietal area on one side. Palpate the vessel and check the direction of blood flow to ensure that a vein and not an artery will be infused. The frontal area may be suitable but avoid the forehead, as extravasation of hypertonic fluids or calcium solutions may leave a scar.

Prepare a 23-gauge butterfly needle by filling it with 0·9% sodium chloride solution. Cut strips of 1·3 cm Micropore tape and 1 × 10 cm gauze impregnated with plaster-of-Paris. For very small veins use a short 25-gauge needle. Make a tourniquet with an elastic band around the head or finger proximal to the site of insertion. Immobilise all but the smallest infants by wrapping the arms in a blanket. Select a Y junction or straight vein. Insert the needle through the skin 0·5 cm before the planned point of entry into the vein, as this distance will help to stabilise the needle. Insert the needle above the vein. Blood should flow back along the tubing. A tiny vein may give very little blood flow but can support a useful infusion for a considerable time.

Place a strip of 1·3 cm Micropore tape on top of the needle. Inject 0·5–1·0 ml of 0·9% sodium chloride solution slowly and check for subcutaneous swelling.

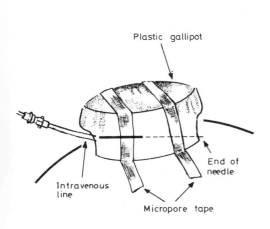

Fixation and immobilisation—If the injection of fluid is satisfactory tape down the wings of the needle and connect the giving set. Check that the fluid flows with gravity. The rate may depend on the tangential angle between the needle and the scalp. Occasionally, flow into a very small vein may be so slow with 0·6–0·9 m of gravity that no flow is visible. Try a test infusion with the pump but beware of extravasation. Plaster-of-Paris gauze or cotton-wool may be packed under the wings to maintain the optimal angle for flow. Plaster-of-Paris gauze may then be spread over the wings, giving effective immobilisation. Tape or plaster a loop of giving set to the scalp.

The butterfly needle should be protected but must be visible to detect extravasation. A plastic cup with two sections cut out gives protection while providing visibility and an exit for the infusion-fluid tube. Tape over the cup securely, covering up to half the head so that the baby can lie on that side. Three or four unsuccessful attempts usually means that you should ask a colleague to try before all the useful veins are spoilt. Don't feel too upset about failure: everyone misses sometimes.

37

SKIN BIOPSY

ALLAN S HIGHET   ROBERT H CHAMPION

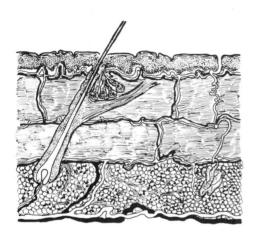

Skin biopsy is an extremely valuable diagnostic technique. The rules are simple, but unless they are followed the results may be disappointing. Histological appearance is the final arbiter in diagnosing few skin disorders. It is not a substitute for clinical assessment but is complementary to it.

The implications of the procedure and the likely consequences (for example, scarring) should be discussed with the patient beforehand.

Aseptic precautions should be similar to those for any other minor surgical procedure.

Preliminary procedure

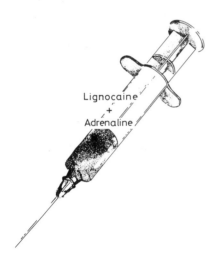

A local anaesthetic is injected just under the skin. Superficial blebs resulting from injecting fluid into the skin itself must be avoided at the biopsy site. Occasionally it is necessary to avoid the biopsy site itself and to inject the anaesthetic in a ring around it—for example, to preserve mast cells.

Vasoconstrictors such as adrenaline and felypressin reduce bleeding but are best avoided in fingers, toes, ears, and penis because intense vasospasm may result in tissue necrosis.

Basic techniques

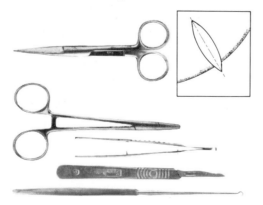

Elliptical excision biopsy—The standard method of skin biopsy is to excise by scalpel an ellipse of skin. Necessary instruments include fine-toothed forceps, needle holder, scalpel, scissors, skin hook, and eyeless needle with suture.

The ellipse should normally measure about 12×4 mm, but smaller specimens may be adequate if required for cosmetic or other reasons. The ends of the ellipse should be pointed to aid closure of the wound. When two specimens are needed from the same site—for example, one for routine histological examination and one for immunofluorescence—two longitudinal halves of the excised ellipse are convenient. It is easier to make the central incision first.

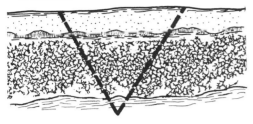

Incorrect

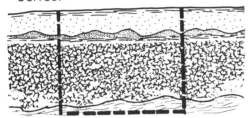

Correct

Incisions should always be made vertical to the skin surface. Incisions slanted inwards result in an unsatisfactory, wedge-shaped specimen and imperfect apposition of the wound edges. The full thickness of skin is incised. The elliptical island of skin, now attached only by the subcutaneous tissue, is lifted by one corner, ideally with a skin hook or needle, and separated, by scalpel or scissors, from the deep tissue to leave attached to the underside of the dermis a thin layer of subcutaneous fat. If pathological changes in the fat are suspected a deeper specimen will be necessary.

Compression by forceps causes tissue distortion. If used at all the forceps should grasp the specimen at one corner only.

Interrupted non-absorbable sutures (for example, silk) are usually used. Equal bites are made on each side of the wound, the needle piercing the skin 2-3 mm from the cut edge. Sutures should be removed after four or five days for the face, 10 days for the leg, and seven days for most other sites. Sometimes adequate closure of the wound may be attained with sterile adhesive tape (Steristrips).

An occlusive dressing kept in place for several days may enhance bacterial growth. The initial dressing should be discarded after a day. If continued cover is desired the dressing should be changed daily.

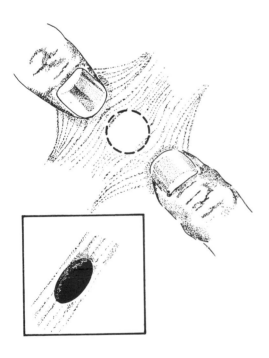

Punch biopsy—The punch is a metal cylinder with a sharp cutting edge at one end. A 6-mm-diameter instrument is preferred for most work, but smaller and larger sizes are available. The punch is pushed with a downward and twisting movement (imparted either by hand or by motor) into the skin, then removed. The specimen is lifted and separated by scissors from the underlying tissue. The wound may be left unsutured or the base cauterised for haemostasis, but inserting one or two stitches gives a better result. Scarring is further minimised by using the punch while traction is applied outwards across the wrinkle lines; when the traction is released the open wound takes up an oval shape.

This method has the advantage of saving time, but most pathologists prefer the elliptical excision method.

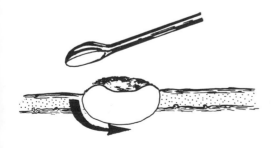

Curettage with a sharp-edged spoon curette followed by cautery may be used to remove certain skin lesions including warts, basal-cell carcinomas seborrhoeic keratoses, and actinic keratoses. Though generally satisfactory for histological examination, curetted specimens are usually incomplete or fragmented (although with care this may be minimised). Curettage, therefore, is mainly a therapeutic procedure and is only indirectly a biopsy technique.

Epidermal (shave) biopsy—Superficial lesions (for example, cellular nae and largely epidermal disorders) may be shaved off by horizontal cutting with a scalpel, the skin being raised if necessary by gentle pinching. The defect may be cauterised for haemostasis.

Needle biopsy—Biopsy needles, like those used for liver biopsy, have been used but are not generally satisfactory.

Skin surface biopsy—A layer of stratum corneum may be removed, attached by adhesive to a glass slide.

Skin biopsy

Choice of site

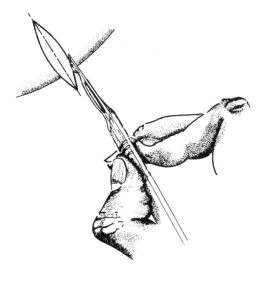

Choice of lesion—In general, a representative lesion at the height of its intensity, unmodified by trauma or treatment, will best show the histological features. The major exceptions are blisters (and pustules), which should be as new as possible and preferably less than a day old when the specimen is taken. An older blister may show confusing changes owing to regeneration, excoriation, or infection.

When the edge of the lesion is well demarcated it is usually best to take the specimen from the edge to include a small portion of normal skin. The edge is often the most active part of the lesion, and the normal skin serves as a built-in control. Sutures often hold better on normal skin. In blistering eruptions, however, perilesional skin is the best site for immunofluorescence and should form the greater proportion of the specimen. When the lesions are poorly demarcated a site of maximum activity should be sought.

Sometimes it may be necessary to take multiple specimens to assess the evolution or varied morphology of lesions.

Orientation of incision—The long axis of the wound should follow the natural wrinkle lines of the skin.

Choice of body site—Some scarring is inevitable, and the site should be chosen to minimise cosmetic disability. With keloids individual predisposition is the main factor, but the chin, midline of the chest, shoulders, and upper outer arms are areas in which the risk of keloid formation is greatest.

Sites subject to much movement, friction, or pressure are best avoided.

Healing on the lower legs is often slow but may be improved by rest and elevation or supportive bandaging.

Skin tumours

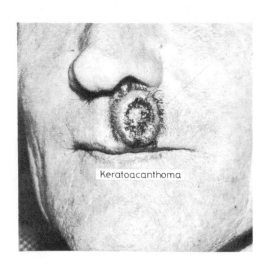

Keratoacanthoma

Suspected malignant melanoma—Clinical diagnosis of malignant melanoma is notoriously inaccurate. A lesion that is strongly suspected of being a melanoma should be widely excised and grafted. When a lesion might only possibly be a melanoma it is better not to inflict such an operation on the patient. The lesion should be completely excised with a minimum margin of 1-2 mm. Further surgery would of course be required should the lesion prove to be a melanoma.

Other malignant tumours—When surgical excision would be the treatment of choice for a suspected malignant tumour direct referral to the surgeon is preferable to a preliminary biopsy.

Keratoacanthoma, a benign, spontaneously regressing tumour, may be histologically confused with squamous carcinoma unless the specimen clearly shows its typical architecture. The specimen should include a segment of the shoulder of the lesion extending into the central crater, along with adjacent normal skin and subcutaneous fat. If the clinical diagnosis of keratoacanthoma can confidently be made curettage, while failing to meet all the above criteria, may be regarded as satisfactory.

Complications

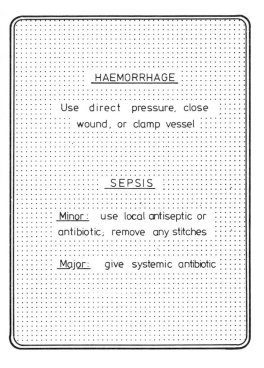

Haemorrhage—Small arteries may be cut, resulting in pulsatile bleeding. This will usually subside spontaneously or respond to direct pressure or wound closure. Occasionally the vessel may have to be clamped and a ligature of absorbable catgut applied.

Scalp incisions may bleed profusely.

Sepsis—Factors predisposing to sepsis include careless technique and occlusive dressings. Minor sepsis responds to a local antiseptic or antibiotic or to removal of stitches when appropriate. Infections with cellulitis, lymphangitis, or lymphadenitis require a systemic antibiotic.

Wounds that gape after infection seldom benefit from resuturing.

Keloids—See above.

What to do with the specimen

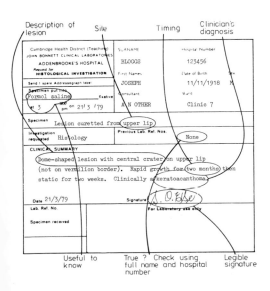

A small specimen may curl. This may be prevented by laying it flat, underside down—that is, epidermis upwards—on a small piece of blotting paper and placing the whole in the fixative. The standard fixative is formol saline.

For examination by immunofluorescence the specimen is preserved by freezing, without chemical fixative. Several techniques are used. In one a 7% gelatin solution (liquefied if necessary by warming) is poured into a small plastic capsule. The specimen is immersed directly in the gelatin and the (labelled) capsule closed and dropped into a flask containing liquid nitrogen. The specimen must remain frozen during transport to the laboratory.

When mast cells are to be examined preliminary fixation is in 70% alcohol. If a specimen has to be cultured for micro-organisms it should not be fixed at all or allowed to dry out. For other special investigations—for example, electron microscopy—the laboratory should be consulted.

The accompanying form must contain adequate identification and a clinical summary including the suspected or differential diagnosis. A sketch of the biopsy area may be helpful. Specimens must, of course, be correctly labelled.

REMOVAL OF DRAINS AND SUTURES

N M KORUTH   PETER F JONES

Reasons for insertion

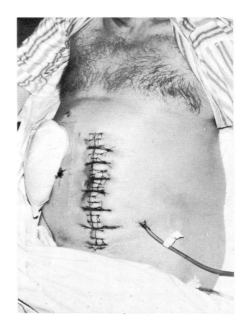

Although drains and sutures are inserted at the end of an operation, when the important parts of the procedure seem to be over, they play an important and at times vital part in the recovery of the patient. It is wise to have a rule that the surgeon who inserted a drain or sutures is the person who decides on removal.

Drains provide a mechanical means of removing material that would otherwise be harmful to the patient, and this may be pus, air, blood, urine, or alimentary secretions. There are three main reasons for inserting drains—namely, to remove air and blood that will delay healing and recovery, to drain abscesses, and to provide a safe and convenient route for secretions to leave the body—and these differing reasons will dictate the way in which the drains are managed.

Removal of air and blood

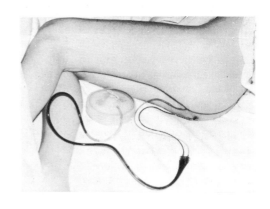

Although in many operations—for instance, inguinal hernia repair—there is no need to insert any drain, in many clean, planned operations considerable areas are opened up. After total mastectomy air is trapped under the skin flaps and blood and serum will, however good the haemostasis, drain from the chest wall and prevent the skin flaps from adhering if drainage is not provided. A haematoma can be dangerous after thyroidectomy and delay healing after excision of the rectum. In all these circumstances efficient drainage is important, but it is equally important that the drain track should provide no entry for bacteria, so a secure system of closed drainage is essential. Most surgeons now use a Redivac type of drain, in which a fine tube with multiple side holes is inserted through a stab wound and attached through closed tubing to a suction bottle: this has proved effective and bacteriologically safe.

The drains are removed when they cease to be useful—usually 24-48 hours after thyroidectomy. After an extensive operation like mastectomy it is important to measure the volume of fluid drained each day, and it is often five to six days before this has dwindled sufficiently to permit removal. These drains are secured by a suture, and on removal this stitch is cut and the drain swiftly withdrawn so that air does not re-enter the wound through the side holes in the tubing.

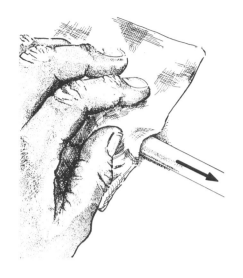

Intrapleural drains require special care because disconnection will result in pneumothorax. All these drains are attached to underwater seal bottles, and, if suction is not being applied to the open end of the bottle, there should be a respiratory swing in the level of fluid in the tubing.

Management of these drains is always under the control of the surgeon. When the drain is ready for removal the suture securing it to the skin is cut, a pad made of a thick square of tulle gras surmounted by several layers of gauze is pressed firmly over wound and drain, and the drain is swiftly withdrawn; the pad is strapped firmly over the drain hole. In this way entry of air into the pleura during removal should be avoided.

Drainage of abscesses and secretions

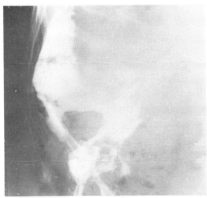

Sometimes drains have to remain in position for a long time. After drainage of a subphrenic abscess or an empyema a large cavity is left, which will contract and heal only slowly: the tube must not be removed until the cavity is obliterated. This process is followed up by injecting sodium diatrizoate (Hypaque) along the drain every seven to 10 days and exposing x-ray plates.

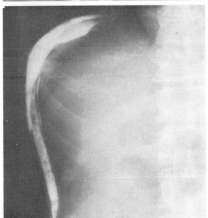

Drains inserted to remove secretions are usually placed in the abdomen. After operations such as cholecystectomy and ureterolithotomy the surgeon hopes that there will be no drainage of bile or urine but cannot be certain of this. Accumulation of bile or urine in the body can cause serious complications, so a soft latex-rubber drainage tube (Sterivac) is placed beside the operation site and attached to a sterile transparent plastic bag. If no appreciable drainage is seen in the bag after 48-72 hours these drains may safely be removed.

When urine is being deliberately diverted through a tube—for example, after suprapubic cystostomy or nephrostomy—the timing of removal depends on the reason for drainage and is decided solely by the operator.

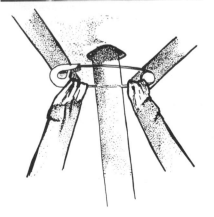

After gastrectomy or intestinal resection and anastomosis there is a period of five to seven days during which the anastomosis is healing but still depends on the integrity of the sutures, so it is essential for the drainage tube beside the anastomosis to remain until this period is over and leakage from the suture line is unlikely. There is always a tendency for fibrinous adhesions to occlude an intraperitoneal drain, so it is wise to shorten such drains after four or five days: this often disturbs adhesions and allows a sealed-off collection of fluid to drain. It is essential to fix the shortened drain securely (use 0·5-in zinc-oxide adhesive tape) so that it cannot be accidentally pulled out.

Removal of drains and sutures

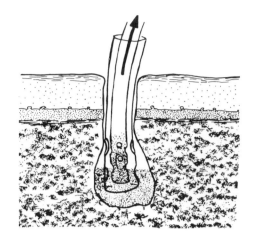

The advantages of using a soft tube instead of corrugated rubber are that the fluid passing along it can be collected, measured, and analysed, and the secretion does not contaminate the abdominal wall. This can be extremely important if, for instance, a pancreatic or small-intestinal fistula should form. Modern disposable drainage bags easily permit collection and measurement and keep the drainage system closed, preventing reflux of air and bacteria along the tubing.

One of the serious aspects of duodenal and pancreatic fistulae is that the enzymes are proteolytic and can cause serious digestion of wounds. With the development of intravenous feeding it is possible to wait while fistulae gradually contract and heal, during which time it is sometimes helpful to use a sump drain. This allows secretions to be aspirated near to their point of origin, which protects the tissues from digestion and keeps the patient comfortable.

Insertion of T tube

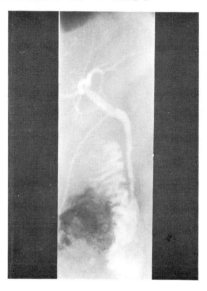

After exploration of the common bile duct a T tube of latex rubber is usually inserted to permit direct drainage of the infected and distended duct. The external end of the tube is placed into a sterile plastic bag (sealed drainage) hanging beside the bed, and the volume of bile drained is recorded every 24 hours: occasionally this volume is high and constitutes an important source of water and electrolyte loss. After eight to 10 days' drainage cholangiography is usually performed to ensure that there is free drainage into the duodenum and no sign of a residual stone. The T tube is withdrawn by steady traction 24 hours later.

Removal of skin sutures

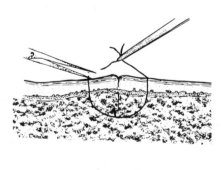

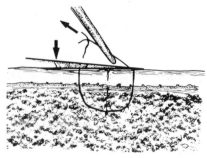

Suture marks—the imprinted scar of the pressure of suture material on the skin surface—are determined by the time for which a suture is left in place, its tension, and its position. The aim must be to remove sutures as soon as their purpose is achieved, and on the face and neck scars heal quickly, so that sutures can usually be removed in 24-72 hours. These sutures are small and fine, and it is essential when removing them to have the patient lying comfortably, to work in a good light, and to have a sharp, fine-pointed pair of scissors and fine, non-toothed dissecting forceps. Always divide the suture close to the skin below the knot and then gently pull the suture out towards the side on which it was divided, using the points of the scissors to give counter pressure on the wound.

Incisions that are made in the line of skin creases heal quickly, and sutures in, for example, an inguinal hernia wound can usually be removed in six or seven days. Vertical abdominal wounds heal more slowly and sutures are removed in seven to 10 days; and sutures in the skin of the back and calf need to remain for 10-12 days. If deep nylon retention sutures are placed in an abdominal wound the surgeon will probably keep them in position for 12-14 days.

INTRAVENOUS UROGRAPHY

BENVON CRAMER   GERALD DE LACEY

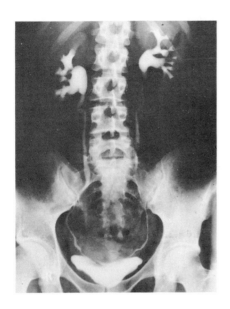

Intravenous urography is the most commonly performed radiological examination of the urinary tract. The information obtained is primarily anatomical, as the examination provides only a crude assessment of renal function. It is, however, highly accurate in delineating the size and shape of the kidneys, calices, and ureters. Most hospitals will have a basic routine procedure, but it must be modified to suit each individual patient. This may entail changing the radiographic technique, dose of contrast medium, and views obtained, and possibly using tomography.

Contraindications

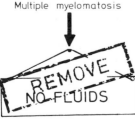

Sensitivity to contrast media

Renal failure

Multiple myelomatosis

Neonates

Pregnancy

Renal failure
Multiple myelomatosis

REMOVE
NO FLUIDS

No absolute contraindications to urography exist but caution should be observed in five groups.

(1) Patients with known sensitivity to radiological contrast media.

(2) Patients with renal failure: transient rises in serum creatinine concentrations after high-dose urography have occurred. Care is particularly important in patients with diabetes mellitus and even mild renal failure.

(3) Patients with multiple myelomatosis.

(4) Neonates.

(5) Pregnant women.

Careful selection is essential in all these patients, and the radiologist will often suggest an alternative and safer procedure such as ultrasonography or isotope renography. For example, when ureteric or bladder-neck obstruction is suspected then ultrasonography will invariably confirm or refute this possibility. When excretion urography is regarded as essential in multiple myeloma or renal failure, however, then the patient should be well hydrated before the procedure. In renal failure dehydration may result in severe volume depletion, electrolyte imbalance, and worsening renal function. Preparing these patients requires more than removing the "no fluids" instruction on the ward. There is often a delay before urography is performed, which can effectively result in a dehydrated patient. It is important that the radiologist and referring clinician make arrangements to see that such inadvertent dehydration does not occur.

The possibility of irradiating an unsuspected fetus is minimised if the x-ray department institutes the "10-day rule"—that is, that women of reproductive age (12-50 years) will be booked for urography only during the first 10 days of their menstrual cycle.

Intravenous urography

Contrast media

Suggested dose of contrast medium according to patient's age and indication

Age and indication	Dose
Adults:	
Routine	50 ml sodium iothalamate (Conray 420)
Renal failure	2 ml meglumine iothalamate (Conray 280)/kg
Children:	
8-12 years	40 ml meglumine iothalamate (Conray 280)
4-8 years	20 ml meglumine iothalamate
< 4 years	2 ml meglumine iothalamate/kg to maximum of 20 ml

The media in use are the sodium and meglumine salts of tri-iodinated organic compounds, which are remarkably safe. Nevertheless, a small risk of hypersensitivity reaction exists and urography should not be undertaken unless equipment and drugs necessary for full resuscitation are readily available. Inquiry about a history of any allergy is always necessary, as the incidence of reactions is increased in atopic patients. Pretesting with small doses of media is now regarded as useless, but in high-risk patients premedication with corticosteroids is necessary, preferably during the 24 hours before the examination.

The choice of contrast medium will vary among radiology departments. There appears to be very little difference in the quality of the x-ray image obtained whether the sodium or meglumine salts are used. In patients with heart failure, however, it is advisable to avoid giving sodium ions (for example, sodium iothalamate (Conray 420)) and therefore to choose instead a meglumine salt (for example, meglumine iothalamate (Conray 280)).

Normal procedure in adults

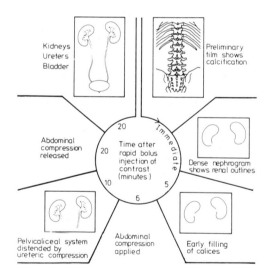

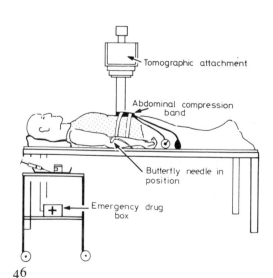

The basic procedure considered here may be modified according to the individual clinical problem. Laxatives are administered for two consecutive nights to remove faeces from overlying the kidneys. Dehydration increases the renal concentration of the contrast medium and improves opacification of the pelvicaliceal systems. Fluids are therefore withheld for 12 hours before urography.

After the patient enters the x-ray department he empties his bladder and a control abdominal film is obtained. This will show opaque calculi and also permits adjustment of the radiographic technique. The patient is always placed supine before the injection of contrast because of the risk of hypotension. In addition he must not be left unattended during the 20 minutes after injection so that any reaction may be detected and treated without delay. Contrast is injected as a rapid bolus to obtain the high serum concentration necessary for a dense nephrogram. A good nephrogram (the radiographic image of the renal parenchyma) shows the outline of the kidneys immediately at the end of the injection. This film reduces the necessity for tomography or oblique views, which might otherwise be required to show the precise outline or size of the kidneys.

A second film is taken five minutes later to show early filling of the calices. Abdominal compression is then applied (though not after recent abdominal surgery, acute abdominal pain, or suspected ureteric colic) to compress the ureters and distend the calices. A further radiograph of the renal areas is obtained at 10 minutes primarily to show the calices and renal pelvis. Compression is released at 20 minutes and a full-length film obtained immediately to show the ureters and bladder. Films of the bladder after micturition are taken only when assessing obstruction of the bladder neck. They are not indicated as a routine procedure, particularly in women.

Procedure in children

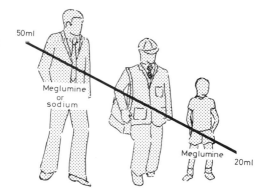

For children, infants, and neonates a different approach is required. The volume of contrast is reduced in relation to body weight, the number of exposures reduced to a minimum, and gonad protection used whenever possible. The clinical indications for urography in neonates are few, and when the procedure is indicated isotopes or ultrasonography will usually and more safely solve the clinical problem. These investigations should precede urography in neonates in most instances.

In children aged under 4 years a meglumine salt is chosen to avoid the hazards of hypernatraemia, and the contrast medium should be injected slowly over several minutes to avoid a sudden rise in plasma osmolarity. In older children eight hours of dehydration suffices and the volume of contrast is reduced.

Special circumstances

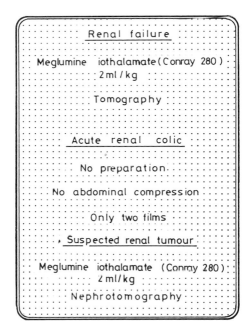

In certain circumstances the standard procedure for intravenous urography must be altered. Renal failure and multiple myeloma have already been mentioned, and the need for careful selection is emphasised. When urography is regarded as essential in renal failure then the dose of contrast medium is increased to 2 ml meglumine iothalamate (Conray 280)/kg and tomography should be routinely available to help delineate the poorly opacified calices and renal parenchyma.

In acute renal colic the investigation is performed without preparation. Abdominal compression is not applied, and two films—a control and a 10-minute film—are often sufficient to confirm or exclude the diagnosis.

When a renal tumour is suspected then a high dose of contrast (for example, 2 ml meglumine iothalamate/kg) with immediate nephrotomography will disclose or exclude a mass and usually distinguish between a simple cyst and a hypernephroma.

Complications

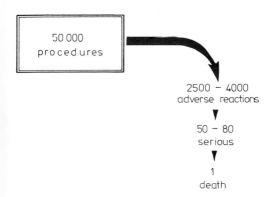

Death due to a reaction to contrast medium is rare, the incidence being about one in 50 000. Adverse reactions of various types and severity occur in 5-8% of patients, but fewer than 2% of these are clinically important. Reactions occur usually within the first 10 minutes after injection but occasionally are delayed. They are mostly mild and include sneezing, pruritus, hives, and minor bronchospasm. When treatment is required an antihistamine, administered intravenously, usually induces a rapid symptomatic response. Severe reactions, including cardiac arrest, are extremely rare but do occur, and the x-ray department must always have facilities and a protocol available for immediate resuscitation.

PROSTATIC BIOPSY

J R RHIND

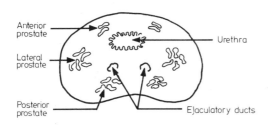

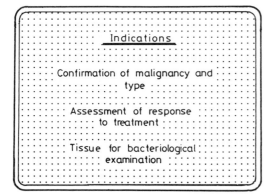

A diagnosis of adenocarcinoma of the prostate based purely on digital examination will be correct in only 70% of cases. Transitional carcinoma may arise in the prostate, as may more rarely sarcoma. The "fibrous prostate," granulomatous prostatitis, and stones may also result in a prostate that feels firmer than normal. Oestrogens or orchidectomy will be of no benefit in these conditions and may cause harm. Histological or cytological proof of the diagnosis is essential.

Examination of prostatic tissue obtained by biopsy has been used to judge the response of a tumour to either hormonal or cytotoxic manipulation. Culture of the prostate may be useful in difficult cases of prostatitis.

Technique

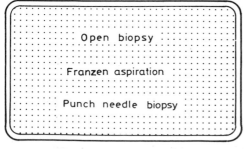

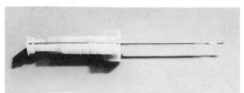

Open biopsy of the prostate by either the perineal or the retropubic route is rarely used in the United Kingdom. Although the perineal approach allows the surgeon the greatest accuracy in obtaining a specimen from a suspicious nodule, the resulting fibrosis may make later total prostatectomy or cystoprostatectomy more difficult. The morbidity is also higher than with the other techniques.

Franzen aspiration of the prostate is the most innocuous of the three techniques but requires the services of a pathologist trained in prostatic cytology and is therefore not always possible.

The most common method of prostatic biopsy practised in the United Kingdom is the punch or needle method using the Tru-Cut needle or the Franklin modification of the Vim-Silverman needle. This provides a core of tissue suitable for routine histological examination.

Method

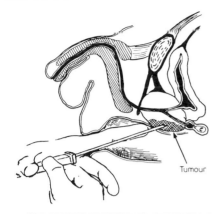

Tumour

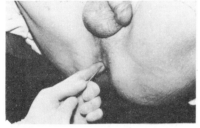

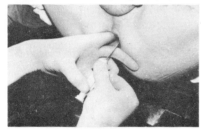

Needle biopsy may be performed as an outpatient procedure, but since penetration of the prostate by the needle causes some discomfort general anaesthesia, local block, or intramuscular pethidine and diazepam are necessary. The patient is placed in either the lithotomy or lateral position with any degree of Trendelenburg thought to be necessary. Very few patients are unsuitable because of ill health or inaccessibility of the prostate.

The biopsy may be performed using either a perineal or a transrectal route; these methods are described separately.

Sampling via the perineal route is a semi-sterile technique and requires the perineum to be shaved and the skin cleansed in the usual manner. A tiny incision in the midline is made with a size 15 blade 1·0–1·5 cm anterior to the anal verge. The biopsy needle is inserted through this incision into the prostate and its course to the area to be sampled estimated by placing a finger in the rectum.

Transrectal biopsy entails passing the needle with the examining finger into the rectum and is therefore a non-sterile technique. To minimise trauma to the anal mucosa the sharp tip of the needle should be protected by the pulp of the finger during insertion. The surgeon then palpates the area of prostate in doubt and the needle is introduced direct through the rectal mucosa.

In both methods tissue is obtained by advancing the trocar and then closing the cannula on to the trocar. With a little practice the trocar may be held firmly by the remaining fingers of the left hand so that removal of the finger from the rectum is not necessary. The tissue is then placed in preservative for histological examination or transport medium for bacteriological examination. Several samples may be obtained at the same time, although this slightly increases the risk of complications.

Complications

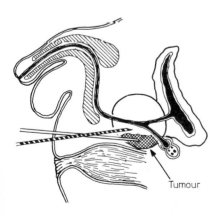

Tumour

```
Biopsy failure
Bleeding
Infection
Tumour implantation
```

Biopsy failure occurs when no tissue is obtained or the histology of the specimen does not agree with the final diagnosis. The transrectal route has a lower failure rate than the perineal route. This is partly because the operator has a better idea of which portion of the prostate the needle is sampling but also because carcinoma tends to arise in the peripheral part of the gland. This area may be missed when the perineal route is used, although with practice the accuracy of this method should improve. Biopsy failure may also occur when the patient has had a prostatectomy so that only the relatively thin shell of the false capsule remains, or when the tissue is so friable that none can be picked up by the needle.

Rectal bleeding or haematuria may occur after biopsy but is only rarely a problem. Haematuria is not uncommon when biopsy is by the perineal route and may persist for several days, but unless the patient has coagulation problems transfusion is unnecessary.

Infection is the main complication of the transrectal route and may proceed to bacteriogenic shock in approximately 0·5% of cases. Prophylactic antibiotics will reduce the infection rate but to be of value must be started before the biopsy procedure.

Tumour implantation is the fear in any biopsy procedure but is extremely rare in the case of prostatic needle biopsy and has been reported only in association with the perineal route.

URETHRAL CATHETERISATION

J T FLYNN   J P BLANDY

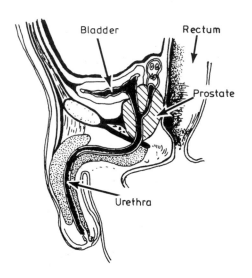

Urethral catheterisation is not to be undertaken lightly and should be performed only by staff who have been properly instructed in the necessary technique. Catheterisation may be used intermittently or continuously, each method having its own specific indications.

Intermittent catheterisation may be (*a*) for diagnostic purposes: either to measure residual urine or to introduce contrast media in radiography of the urinary tract; or (*b*) for therapeutic purposes: in the hypotonic, neurogenic, or decompensated bladder to permit adequate emptying, especially when managing chronic urinary infection.

Continuous catheterisation may be short term to relieve acute or chronic retention of urine before prostatectomy, or long term when general poor health prevents prostatectomy (rarely) or mental deterioration and urinary incontinence make a permanent indwelling catheter the most acceptable method of treatment.

Catheters

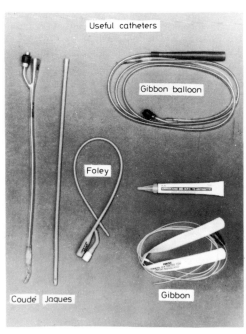

Which catheter you put in depends on what you expect to get out. When you expect the urine to be clear and do not have to leave the catheter in afterwards you should use the softest, narrowest, and cheapest catheter available. The disposable Jaques catheter is quite suitable for this purpose. Indwelling catheters are usually retained by a balloon and should be biologically inert to prevent urethral irritation. Latex is usually well tolerated, and the newer polyvinylchloride catheters are said to be non-irritant.

When blood clot or debris has to be washed out use a plastic or armoured latex catheter, as this will not collapse when suction is applied. If irrigation of the bladder is required a three-channel catheter should be used, but remember that the third channel narrows the lumen of the catheter.

In retention a small Foley catheter of 12-14 French gauge will usually be suitable, but in men with a large prostate or prominent bladder neck a smaller (8-10 French gauge) Gibbon catheter, which is more resilient, will often go in more easily. For long-term drainage a larger catheter (18-20 French gauge) made of silicone rubber should be used. These catheters are said to be more comfortable and require less frequent changing as fewer encrustations develop.

50

Procedure in men

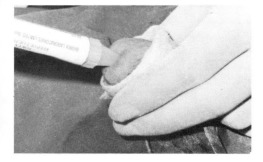

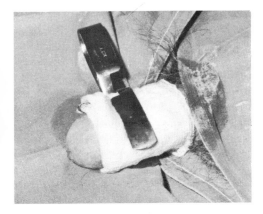

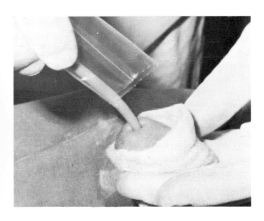

Absolute asepsis in technique, adequate light, and the utmost care in passing the catheter are essential. The patient should be resting comfortably on his back on a table or bed, with his legs separated slightly to accommodate the sterile receptacle for the urine collection. Explain to the patient what you are about to do and reassure him. Use sedation if necessary. Gloves and mask should be worn: this will remind everyone that it is an aseptic procedure and will keep it so should you have to change catheters or use an introducer.

The prepuce (if present) is fully retracted and, together with the glans and separated meatus, thoroughly cleansed with an antiseptic solution—for example, 0·5% aqueous chlorhexidine. Sterile drapes are placed around the penis, which is wrapped in a sterile gauze swab soaked in the antiseptic solution. This makes the penis easier to hold and keeps the foreskin retracted during the procedure.

A gel (15 ml) containing 1% lignocaine and 0·5% chlorhexidine is introduced into the urethra and retained for five minutes by using a sterile penile clamp. The lignocaine anaesthetises the urethra and lubricates it for passage of the catheter. Chlorhexidine inhibits the growth of any bacteria carried into the urethra and bladder by the catheter. (*Note*: lignocaine is absorbed through the mucosa and should not be used in quantities of more than 15 ml or strengths greater than 1%.)

It is useful at this point to check that you have all that you require on the catheter trolley. The time spent doing this will allow the lignocaine to work and ensure a smooth catheterisation.

The catheter may be handled by the gloved hand, or advanced in a no-touch technique by using the inner polyethylene sheath in which the catheter is packed or two pairs of forceps. The penis should be slightly stretched with the opposite hand to straighten out mucosal folds. No force should be used at any time.

Usually there is a little resistance to the catheter when its tip meets the external sphincter. It may help if the patient takes a deep breath, for as he breathes out the catheter can usually be gently pushed through the sphincter. Occasionally a prominent middle lobe of prostate or bladder neck will obstruct the catheter, and a curved catheter (coudé) or introducer may be necessary to get over the hump. Introducers should be used only by medical staff properly trained in urethral instrumentation, as great damage to the urethra may result from inexpert manipulation with one. It is important to lubricate the introducer before inserting it into the catheter, and to check that the tip is well engaged in the blunt tip of the catheter.

The balloon of the catheter is inflated with the appropriate volume of sterile water, and a specimen of urine is collected in a sterile container for bacteriological studies. Finally, the catheter is connected to a closed drainage system, thereby reducing the chance of subsequent infection. Remember to advance the foreskin at the end of the procedure to prevent the development of a paraphimosis.

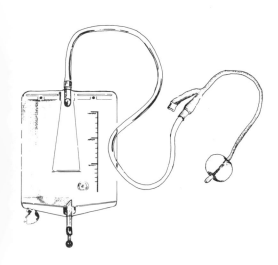

Failure may be due to the presence of a urethral stricture or spasm of the external sphincter. If a small Gibbon catheter cannot be easily passed, more expert help should be sought.

Urethral catheterisation

Procedure in women and children

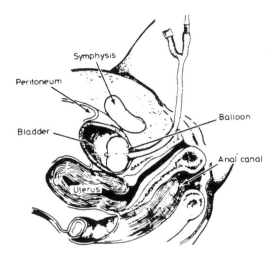

Symphysis

Peritoneum

Balloon

Bladder

Anal canal

Uterus

In women catheterisation is often performed by nurses, who should be taught the necessary technique. A good light is essential, as the urethral meatus tends to become more vaginal in postmenopausal, sexually inactive women and is occasionally difficult to find. The bladder neck is sometimes prominent and may be passed by directing the catheter tip slightly anteriorly.

Children require careful handling and may be helped by sedation. A small Gibbon catheter or infant feeding tube is often the most useful. Balloon catheters tend to produce bladder spasm and are not always well tolerated.

Aftercare and complications

Aftercare

Catheter toilet

Maintenance of closed
drainage system

Maintenance of free drainage

Regular examination of catheter
specimen of urine

Complications

Infection

False passage

Haemorrhage

Blocked catheter

Organisms can enter the urinary tract from three sources once a catheter has been left indwelling: (*a*) by retrograde spread from urine in the reservoir; (*b*) by a break in the closed drainage system; and (*c*) from bacterial colonisation of the urethral meatus. Growth of bacteria in the reservoir bag may be prevented by introducing antiseptic into the bag. Breaks in the closed drainage system usually occur when the catheter is irrigated because of blood clot. It is essential that this is done aseptically, otherwise infection will certainly follow. Bacterial colonisation of the urethral meatus may be reduced by regular catheter toilet—that is, by cleansing the glans and adjacent catheter with antiseptic.

Traumatic catheterisation with rupture of the urethra and the catheter tip placed outside the urethra or bladder will result in extravasation of urine with tissue necrosis and gangrene if unrecognised. This is a surgical emergency and requires expert surgical help. The complications of infection and bacteraemia are difficult to eliminate, but good aseptic techniques and careful monitoring of ward infections will help to reduce their incidence.

SETTING UP A DRIP

BARBARA BANNISTER   C W H HAVARD

Indications

The many indications for setting up a drip fall into three main groups.

(1) To introduce or replace fluids into the circulation—for example, blood, blood fractions, colloids, or electrolyte solutions.

(2) To provide a route for administering parenteral medication or nutrition, usually in intensive care.

(3) To permit monitoring of central venous pressures: in this case a long flexible catheter is used to reach along the peripheral vein into the vena cava.

Precautions

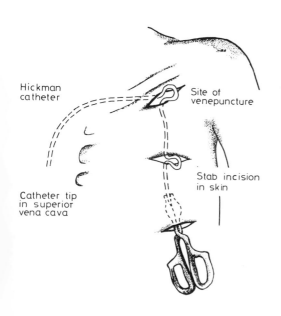

No absolute contraindications exist, but particular care is neccessary under some circumstances.

(1) If heart failure is present or incipient an extra circulating fluid load may result in severe pulmonary oedema. If a blood transfusion or intravenous infusion is essential this problem may be alleviated by giving diuretics simultaneously.

(2) In renal failure it is important that the fluid and electrolyte loads, as well as the amount of drugs given, do not exceed the excretory capabilities of the kidneys.

(3) If small veins with inadequate blood flow are cannulated toxic or irritant substances may pool at the infusion site, causing inflammation or necrosis.

(4) In patients with impaired immune responses or damaged heart valves a drip site is an important portal for the entry of potentially fatal infection. Strict attention to asepsis and restriction of the time for which the cannula is in situ are necessary. If prolonged use of a long catheter is expected the outer end should be drawn through a skin "tunnel," so that the site of the skin puncture is several centimetres from the vein—for example, Broviac or Hickman catheters. The stab wounds are closed with a stitch when the catheter is in position, and the giving-set connection is outside the tunnel, strapped to the chest wall.

Setting up a drip

Equipment

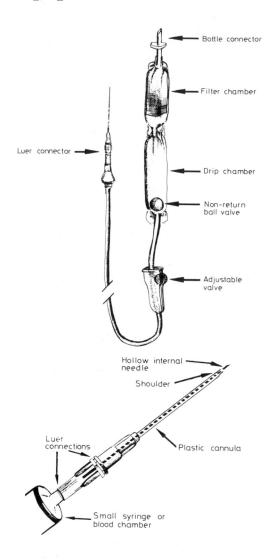

Sterile fluid and giving set—The fluid or blood is usually presented in collapsible bags or bottles, but it is sometimes in rigid bottles, which need an air inlet to prevent a vacuum from forming when the fluid flows out into the giving set. To prepare the giving set close the adjustable valve before pushing the connector firmly into the bag or bottle outlet. Squeeze the drip chamber to obtain a fluid level in it. Raise the Luer connector, with its sterile cover, above the fluid level and open the valve. The fluid will fill the plastic tubing up to the level in the drip chamber, and by lowering the Luer connector to that level the whole tubing will be filled, without the formation of bubbles. Any small bubbles will float to the fluid surfaces if the tube is held vertical and tapped sharply. Turn off the valve; the set is ready for use.

Cannulae (for example, Medicut, Venflon, Abbocath)—Long catheters are flexible plastic or silicon, with radio-opaque markers. They are passed through previously inserted metal or plastic cannulae, which are withdrawn from the skin after use. Great care must be taken when inserting catheters through metal cannulae, as the sharp needle may sever the catheter if it is accidentally withdrawn. The severed part may then embolise to the heart or lung. Care is also needed to insert long catheters with a suitable sterile technique. Detailed instructions are provided and should be studied before the procedure is begun.

Procedure

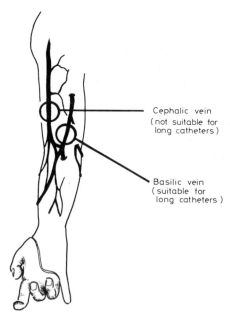

Choice of vein—The most convenient site is the left forearm (or the right in a left-handed patient). This permits comfortable mobility of the left arm and leaves the right free for writing, washing, etc. Veins at the elbow should be avoided, as the joint would then require immobilisation to avoid repeated kinking of the cannula or catheter with resulting fracture and leakage. The site may, however, be dictated by the availability of suitable veins. Leg veins may be used in restless patients, as it is easier to splint a dressing on the leg than the arm. The experienced operator may cannulate the jugular, subclavian, or saphenous vein, or a scalp vein in a baby. Veins are much easier to cannulate at a site where they penetrate fascia, or at a confluence, as they are then fixed and cannot roll sideways away from the needle point. The cephalic vein is extremely difficult to cannulate with a long catheter, since it is angled at the shoulder; the basilic vein is much easier.

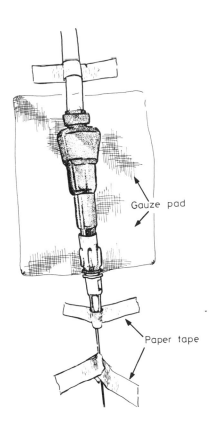

Gauze pad

Paper tape

Venepuncture—After clothes have been removed from the limb a tourniquet should be applied to distend the veins. Careful sterile procedure is important; a generous area around the chosen site should be cleaned with isopropyl alcohol swabs or iodine in alcohol solution. Heavy hair growth should be shaved before this is done. When long catheters are to be used sterile drapes and gloves make the procedure easier and safer. The needle and cannula should first be inserted through the skin, beyond the shoulder of the plastic part. The metal needle is then adjusted until it is touching the vein, with the flat side of the bevel pointing to the surface. Sharp oblique pressure causes the bevel to enter the vein, and pressure is continued until the plastic shoulder of the cannula has followed. Blood will then enter the chamber or may be drawn into the syringe. The metal needle is then withdrawn from the cannula, while leakage of blood is prevented by pressing the finger on the vein over the tip of the cannula; the giving set is connected and the tourniquet removed.

Fixing and dressing—The cannula must be fixed securely, as movement may damage it and lead to leakage and inflammation. A crêpe bandage may be applied overall and helps to warm the fluid as it flows towards the vein. Splints should be avoided if possible, as movement of the limb discourages stasis of blood and possible thrombosis.

The site should be examined daily for inflammation, as a skin puncture always allows micro-organisms to enter the tissues and hypertonic glucose and amino-acid solutions are excellent culture media. Adding 500 units of heparin to each 500 ml of fluid infused reduces the incidence of catheter-associated sepsis. All short cannulae should be resited at two- or three-day intervals before infection reaches the circulation. Giving sets should be removed after three or four days and immediately after a blood transfusion, as clot remains in the filter chamber and may harbour micro-organisms.

Problems

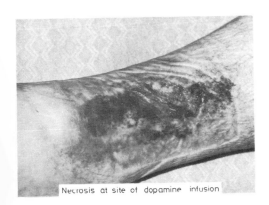

Necrosis at site of dopamine infusion

No veins are visible or pulpable—A "cut-down" technique may be performed: a vein is exposed by blunt dissection of subcutaneous tissues through a small incision and is cannulated under direct vision. Alternatively, an experienced operator may cannulate the subclavian or jugular vein.

Failure to penetrate the vein—This is common when elderly patients have fibrous or calcified veins. Remove the tourniquet and apply pressure to the venepuncture site in case the vein is leaking. Anaesthetists do many venepunctures and may succeed when all others have failed.

Failure to flow—Check that the tourniquet has been removed, that the giving-set valve is open, and that rigid bottles have an adequate air inlet. The appearance of a large bleb of subcutaneous fluid shows that the cannula is not in the vein lumen and should be resited. Finally, the cannula should be vigorously flushed with fluid in case it is blocked by a clot.

Appearance of inflammation—The cannula must be resited, as local antiseptics or systemic antibiotics will be useless while a foreign body is in position. The cause of unexplained fever in the patient may be infection at the venepuncture site.

Careful attention to siting, dressing, and managing a drip can make the difference between wellbeing and misery for the patient, and is very rewarding for the little time that it takes.

HORMONE IMPLANTATION

MARGARET H THOM   J W W STUDD

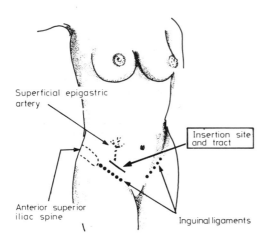

Superficial epigastric artery

Insertion site and tract

Anterior superior iliac spine

Inguinal ligaments

The implantation of pellets of oestradiol into the fat of the abdominal wall or buttock has been used for 30 years, mainly to treat young patients who have undergone hysterectomy and bilateral oophorectomy. More recently its use has been extended to patients with an intact uterus, and potential complications of endometrial hyperplasia and heavy vaginal bleeding are avoided by adding a seven- to 13-day course of a progestogen each month.

Indications

Indications

Symptoms of climacteric

No gonadal androgens

Contraindications

Endometrial and breast carcinoma

Deep vein thrombosis

Pulmonary embolus

Emotional instability

Treatment of the climacteric—Subcutaneous hormone implants are principally used to treat the symptoms of the climacteric. When classic symptoms such as hot flushes, sweats, insomnia, vaginal dryness, and dyspareunia predominate a pellet of oestradiol 50 mg may be sufficient. Adding testosterone 100 mg to the oestradiol pellet, however, is effective in treating the related climacteric symptoms of loss of libido, lethargy, and depression. The sense of wellbeing induced by the anabolic effect of testosterone is considerable. There are obvious contraindications such as the presence or history of endometrial or breast carcinoma and a history of deep vein thrombosis or pulmonary embolus. It is also unwise to insert hormone pellets in emotionally unstable patients, who after implantation are apt to focus all anxieties on the pellets and request their removal soon after insertion.

Male hormone replacement—The rare patients with no gonadal androgen production—for example, after surgery—may be treated by implanting testosterone. A minimum of 1 g is required, necessitating the insertion of 10 pellets. Therefore, sufficient subcutaneous fat to accommodate these is an advantage. The possible hepatotoxic effects of the oral 17-alkylated androgen methyltestosterone are thus avoided.

Non-hormonal use in alcoholism—Pellets of disulfiram (Antabuse) are now available and may be implanted into patients suffering from alcoholism who cannot be relied on to take oral treatment consistently.

Procedure

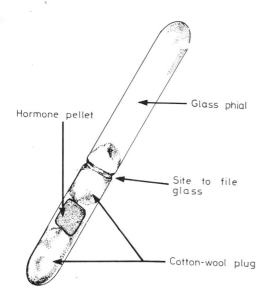

Hormone pellet

Glass phial

Site to file glass

Cotton-wool plug

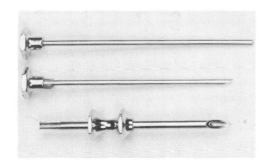

Implantation is performed as an outpatient procedure during a routine clinic visit and never necessitates admission to hospital or general anaesthesia. A no-touch technique and sterile instruments are used. Scrubbing-up is not necessary.

The anterior abdominal wall, 5 cm above and parallel to the inguinal ligament, is the commonest site chosen for insertion. A small area of skin around the site is cleaned with iodine, spirit, or any antiseptic. About 2-5 ml of 1% lignocaine is drawn up and the skin and subcutaneous tissues of the insertion site infiltrated. During the minute or so required for effective anaesthesia the sterilised trocar and cannula may be assembled and the obturator placed alongside in a sterile dish ready for use.

A file is used to scratch the glass phial containing the hormone pellet. The phial is broken, allowing the pellet to fall into a sterile gallipot. A sterile No 11 surgical blade, a pair of sterile forceps, some sterile cotton-wool, and two Band-Aids must also be at hand. The pointed blade is used to make a 4-5 mm incision in the skin over the insertion point. This incision does not have to be deep, as it is needed only to ease the passage of the pointed trocar and cannula through the firm skin. The trocar and cannula are then pushed through the incision as far as possible into the fat, avoiding the rectus sheath and muscle and any scar from previous surgery.

The trocar is withdrawn and the gallipot containing the pellets held under the cannula opening. The pellets are then placed in the cannula by using sterile forceps with the gallipot held under the cannula: in this way expensive pellets do not fall and become unsterile. The obturator is inserted into the cannula, forcing the pellets out of the instrument medial to the insertion site. Two cotton-wool balls are then placed over the insertion site and the tract as the obturator and cannula are simultaneously withdrawn. Slight pressure is kept on the cotton-wool for at least a minute by the operator, preventing any minor bleeding. The Band-Aid plasters are then placed over the wound. The patient is advised to keep the dressing dry for 48 hours.

When the buttock is chosen the site of insertion is that used for intramuscular injections but the tract is kept in the subcutaneous tissues.

Implantation of pellets will usually be repeated when symptoms return after six to nine months.

Complications

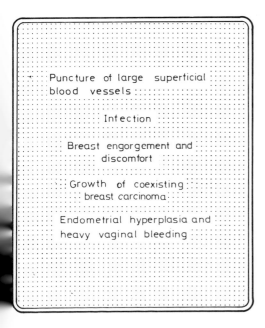

Puncture of large superficial blood vessels

Infection

Breast engorgement and discomfort

Growth of coexisting breast carcinoma

Endometrial hyperplasia and heavy vaginal bleeding

(1) Difficulty may be encountered in pushing the trocar and cannula through tough skin, and deepening the incision with a surgical blade may help.

(2) The site of insertion should be chosen to avoid any large superficial blood vessels.

(3) Haemostasis may be difficult to secure if a small vessel has been punctured. Prolonged manual pressure over the wound is required and, rarely, a stitch for a skin bleeder. Pressure over the tract prevents subsequent haematoma formation, but the patient will probably have an area of bruising around the wound the following day.

(4) Infection should be rare if a no-touch technique is adhered to. If it occurs the pellets may be extruded.

(5) Prolonged breast engorgement and discomfort are symptoms of oestrogen overdosage.

(6) Oestrogens may promote growth of a coexisting breast carcinoma. If breast carcinoma is diagnosed during the course of treatment it is advisable to remove the pellets.

(7) Endometrial hyperplasia and heavy vaginal bleeding may occur if the patient omits to take her seven to 13 days of progestogen each month.

Hormone implantation

Hormone profiles after implantation

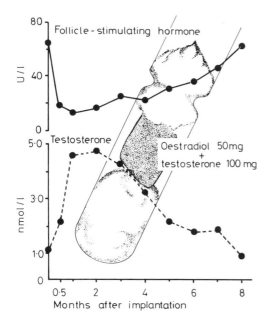

The depression of plasma concentrations of follicle-stimulating hormone by the 50 mg of oestradiol used in treating the climacteric is dramatic and prolonged. The concentrations fall to premenopausal values of 15 IU/l within two weeks of implantation, where they remain for up to six months. The 50 mg oestradiol pellet causes mean plasma oestradiol concentrations of 320 pmol/l (87 pg/ml) and oestrone concentrations of 230 pmol/l (62 pg/ml) eight weeks after implantation. These are comparable with the concentrations found in the normal luteal phase of the cycle and may be contrasted with the abnormally high concentrations of oestrone found after oral oestrone or oestradiol treatment.

After implantation of 100 mg testosterone plasma testosterone concentrations rise from 1 to 5 nmol/l (0·3 to 1·4 ng/ml) after six weeks, when the patient reports symptomatic improvement of energy and libido problems. Testosterone has no effect on plasma concentrations of follicle-stimulating hormone. Hirsutism is not a problem with the dose of testosterone used.

Prevention of hyperplasia

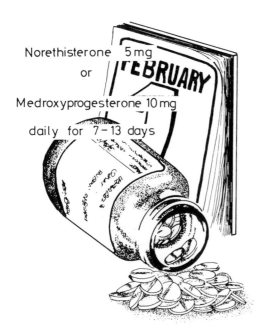

Implanting hormones in patients who have had a hysterectomy is straightforward, but there is a risk of endometrial hyperplasia if a regular course of progestogen is not taken by patients with a uterus. We prescribe seven to 13 days of a progestogen each month in the form of 5 mg norethisterone daily or 10 mg medroxyprogesterone. It is convenient for this progestogen course to start on the first day of each calendar month, and bleeding occurs two days after taking the last tablet.

Patients may feel unpleasant symptoms of breast discomfort, depression, headaches, and bloatedness with the progestogen, and a few may omit taking this regular course in an attempt to avoid these symptoms or, misguidedly, to avoid having periods altogether. In these patients a period of amenorrhoea will be followed by heavy bleeding owing to hyperplasia. This should be investigated by curettage, and the hyperplasia may be corrected by two or three courses of progestogen for 21 days each month.

PERICARDIAL ASPIRATION

R J WARRELL   R W PORTAL

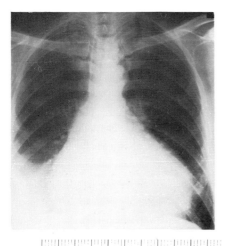

Pericardial aspiration is seldom indicated, and many doctors will neither have witnessed the procedure during training nor have performed it later in their careers. It is a potentially hazardous procedure and should not be performed except in emergencies unless facilities for resuscitation are available. Before inserting a needle into the pericardium there must be good evidence that an effusion is present.

Diagnosis of effusion

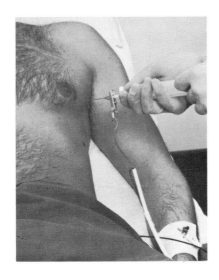

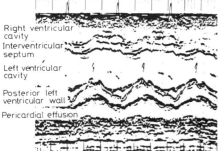

Right ventricular cavity

Interventricular septum

Left ventricular cavity

Posterior left ventricular wall

Pericardial effusion

Clinical signs—Clues on examination may or may not be present. Three indications are pulsus paradoxus, in which the pulse pressure diminishes during inspiration and increases during expiration; raised jugular venous pressure on inspiration (Kussmaul's sign); and muffled heart sounds.

Chest x-ray films—In acute tamponade (for example, haemorrhage from trauma) the chest film may show little or no cardiac enlargement. When time has permitted stretching of the pericardium the cardiac silhouette may be grossly enlarged and appear pear-shaped with bulging over the right atrium and apex.

Echocardiography is the most reliable method of proving a pericardial effusion, but the results require skilled interpretation. The ultrasonic beam shows a space between the pericardium and the anterior right or posterior left ventricular wall.

Cardiac catheterisation and angiography are no longer justifiable for showing an effusion.

Pericardial aspiration

Indications

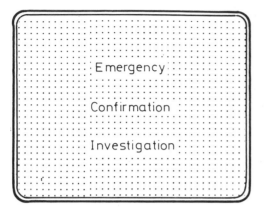

(1) As an emergency procedure to relieve cardiac tamponade.

(2) To confirm the presence of a pericardial effusion. The availability of echocardiography in most centres has rendered the procedure unnecessary for this purpose.

(3) To obtain samples of pericardial fluid for analysis—for example, culture, cytology.

Routes

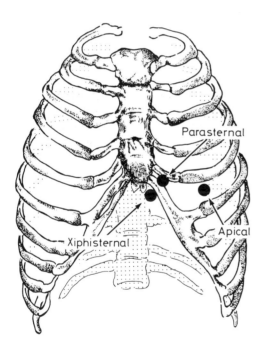

Xiphisternal route—The safest route is through the angle between the xiphoid process and the left costal margin. The needle is aimed upward at an angle of 45° to the skin and backward towards the spine between the scapulae. The needle passes through the membranous portion of the diaphragm and enters the pericardium at the inferior surface of the heart over the right ventricle.

Apical route—The needle is introduced at the cardiac apex in the fourth or fifth intercostal space 2 cm medial to the lateral edge of cardiac dullness. It is aimed at right angles to the skin (that is, slightly medially) and slightly upward. This route carries a greater risk of injury to the coronary arteries and contamination of the pleural space when the pericardial fluid is purulent.

Parasternal route—The needle is introduced in the fifth left intercostal space just to the left of the sternum and aimed straight backward. The internal mammary artery lies about 2 cm lateral to the sternal edge and the needle must pass medial to this: laceration of the artery is the main complication of this route.

Procedure

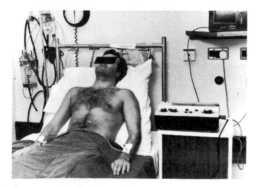

The patient should be undressed to the waist and sitting comfortably in bed at an angle of 45°. He should be connected to an electrocardiograph (ECG) or monitor, and an intravenous line should be inserted for administering drugs. A gown, gloves, and a mask should be worn. The patient's chest should be cleaned with an antiseptic solution —for example, iodine—and a sterile towel positioned across his abdomen and legs. An 18-gauge lumbar-puncture needle is used, connected to a 30-ml syringe via a three-way tap. A sterilised length of wire with an "alligator" clip at each end is used to connect the needle to the V lead of the ECG.

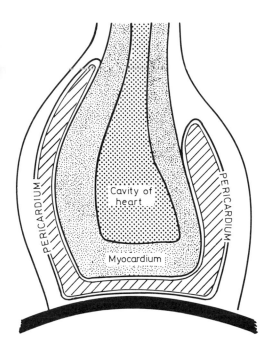

The skin and deep tissues in the direction of the route to be used are infiltrated with 10 ml of lignocaine 2%. The needle is introduced and advanced slowly, aspiration being carried out at frequent intervals, until the pericardial sac is entered and fluid, if present, is drawn into the syringe. If the needle is advanced too far the myocardium will be felt knocking against the tip or will cause the needle to waggle. If this occurs, withdraw the needle—never advance it further.

A pair of Spencer-Wells forceps is then clamped to the needle next to the skin to prevent further inadvertent penetration. By using the syringe and three-way tap fluid is aspirated; samples are sent for culture, cytology, and so on.

A bloody effusion may be distinguished from blood aspirated from the heart by placing a sample in a glass specimen bottle. A bloody effusion will not clot.

In cases in which repeated aspiration may be necessary a large needle may be used and a soft plastic cannula passed through this. The needle is then withdrawn, leaving the cannula in the pericardial space.

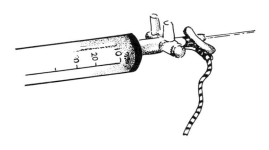

The ECG—The monitor attached to the needle will show a complex like the normal V1 complex until the needle comes into contact with the heart. Contact with the ventricle may cause an injury pattern with ST elevation to appear. Contact with the myocardium may cause ectopic beats, which may be atrial or ventricular in origin depending on the area of the heart that has been touched.

Complications

Vasovagal reaction (bradycardia, hypotension) may occur after entry of the needle into the pericardium.

Laceration of a coronary artery.

Laceration of the left internal mammary artery.

Laceration of the ventricle wall.

Laceration of the lung.

Spread of infection locally from a purulent effusion.

Arrhythmias.

PLEURAL ASPIRATION AND BIOPSY

P B ILES   COLIN OGILVIE

Indications

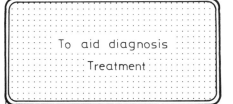

To aid diagnosis

Treatment

Pleural aspiration may be needed for diagnosis or treatment.

Diagnosis—To confirm that there is effusion (rather than consolidation or collapse); to diagnose empyema and haemothorax; to distinguish transudate from exudate by the protein content; and to identify malignancy and infection by cytological examination and culture.

Treatment—To relieve dyspnoea; to remove blood or pus; and to instil antibiotics for empyema.

Aspiration procedure

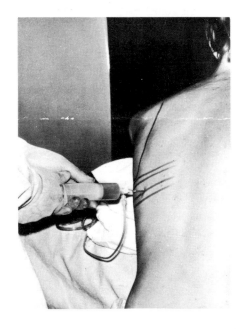

Fluid analysis

Microscopy: blood-cell type, tumour cells, organisms

Bacteriological culture including *Mycobacterium tuberculosis*

Biochemical measurement: protein + glucose concentrations

It is important that the patient is as comfortable and relaxed as possible; some explanation of what he will feel during the procedure should be given. The best site for pleural aspiration is decided by locating the fluid by percussion and from posteroanterior and lateral radiographs. A common error in cases of difficulty is to insert the needle too low down or too far forward. When the fluid is not loculated the easiest site for puncture is on the posterior chest wall medial to the angle of the scapula. The patient should be positioned leaning slightly forwards with his arms folded comfortably before him and resting on a pillow. He may be either seated facing the side of his bed with his arms on it or in bed with a bed table as support for his arms.

The operator should scrub up and be gloved and gowned as for any surgical procedure. The patient's skin is prepared with a suitable antiseptic and sterile towels. The skin overlying an intercostal space at the chosen level is infiltrated with 1% or 2% lignocaine using a 25-gauge (orange-hub) needle. This is then changed for a 21-gauge needle (green hub) to infiltrate the chest wall down to the pleura. When the needle penetrates the pleura fluid should appear in the syringe as the plunger is withdrawn. To avoid damaging the intercostal neurovascular bundle the inferior border of the upper rib is avoided. Care must be taken to ensure that air does not enter the pleural space at any stage of the procedure.

When the tap is for diagnosis only, 20-50 ml fluid is aspirated into a fresh sterile syringe and put into sterile plastic or glass containers. These are labelled and sent for microscopy for blood cells, cytology, and organisms; for bacterial culture (including acid-fast bacilli); and for estimations of protein, fat (if chylous), and glucose content (low in rheumatoid disease).

To remove a large quantity of fluid use a needle with attached three-way tap or a ready-prepared pack consisting of needle, three-way tap, connecting plastic tubing, syringe, and collecting bag. Aspirating large volumes of fluid in this manner may be protracted and uncomfortable for the patient, and it is sometimes easier to insert a catheter such as the 12- or 14-gauge E-Z Cath intravenous placement unit and, after withdrawing the central needle and stylet, to connect a three-way tap and syringe to the Luer fitting on the end. When the needle or catheter is removed a small adhesive dressing is adequate for the puncture site.

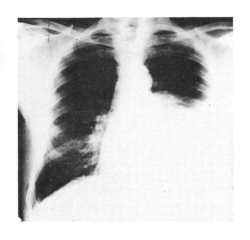

Patients with empyema and haemothorax—Difficulties may arise in patients with empyema and haemothorax when the fluid is thick or loculated. Aspiration may be possible only with a large-bore needle, and exploratory aspiration at several different sites may be necessary. The finding of pus is an indication for instilling antibiotics while the needle is in the empyema space; it may be difficult to locate the space at a later attempt. If the empyema is a complication of a bacterial pneumonia then laboratory information on the organism and its antibiotic sensitivities may already be available to guide the choice of antibiotic. If this guidance is not available then ampicillin (500-1000 mg) in 10-20 ml of water for injection or a cephalosporin should be instilled. Foul-smelling pus usually indicates an anaerobic infection, for which metronidazole is appropriate. Repeated aspiration and intrapleural instillation of antibiotic should be continued until pus is no longer obtainable. If there is then still evidence of continuing infection insertion of an intercostal drainage tube is indicated, followed, if necessary, by rib resection with evacuation of the empyema cavity.

Biopsy equipment

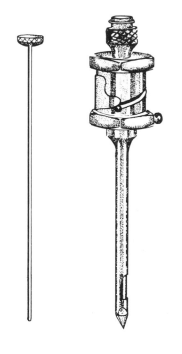

Needle biopsy of the pleura should be performed at the time of diagnostic pleural aspiration if the cause of the effusion is not then apparent. If mesothelioma is strongly suspected, however, it is better to avoid needle biopsy because of the risk of seeding mesothelioma cells in the needle track. Fluid cytology without biopsy is sometimes sufficient for diagnosing this condition.

The Abrams needle is the one most widely used in Britain for pleural biopsy. The blunt-type Cope needle may be more suitable when little or no pleural fluid is present. The Abrams needle consists of outer and inner tubes, the outer acting as a trocar. Behind the tip of the outer tube is an opening into which a fold of pleura is to be impacted. This opening is closed completely when the cutting edge of the inner tube is advanced by twisting its hexagonal grip clockwise. This rotation moves a pin in the hilt of the inner tube forwards along a spiral slot in the hilt of the outer tube. The biopsy specimen is cut by the advancing edge of the inner tube and is retained within the instrument. It can then be retrieved by using the accompanying blunt obturator.

Biopsy procedure

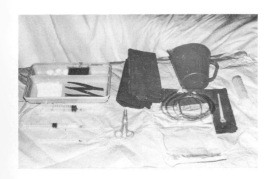

Position and prepare the patient as for a pleural tap, and infiltrate the intercostal tissues at the chosen site with lignocaine. Make a short incision (3-5 mm) through the skin and deeper tissues with a sharp, pointed scalpel blade; the closed Abrams needle is then introduced through the tissues and parietal pleura with a slight rotary movement. Connect a three-way tap and syringe to the Luer fitting on the needle, rotate the hexagonal hub of the inner tube anticlockwise to open the notch, and aspirate pleural fluid in the usual manner. The needle is airtight when the notch is closed, but a syringe or closed three-way tap must be attached when the notch is open to prevent air entering the pleural cavity.

Pleural aspiration and biopsy

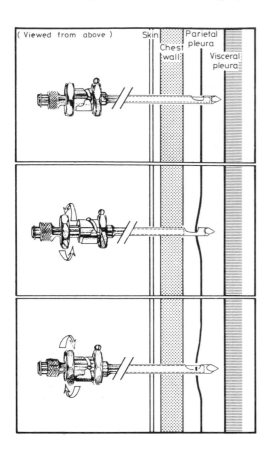

When taking a biopsy specimen it is convenient to have a small (2 ml) syringe attached to the needle. Rotate the grip to open the notch, which faces the same direction as the spherical marker on one facet of the hexagonal base of the outer tube. With this marker (and therefore the notch) facing along the line of the intercostal space (to the left if the operator is right-handed), apply lateral pressure towards the notch with the forefinger and slowly withdraw the needle until resistance is felt owing to pleura catching in the notch. If the needle is withdrawn too far only intercostal muscle will be obtained. Hold the needle firmly and sharply twist the grip of the inner tube clockwise to take the specimen. Withdraw the needle with a slight rotary action when the patient exhales. To avoid damage to the intercostal neurovascular bundle the notch should never be directed upwards. The specimen will be found either within the inner tube or in the tip of the needle and should be put in 10% formol saline. If tuberculous pleurisy is suspected a second pleural biopsy specimen should be taken and placed in a dry sterile container for bacteriological culture.

Complications of pleural aspiration and biopsy

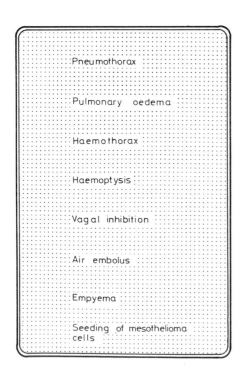

If fluid is removed too quickly or in too great a quantity oedema may develop in the re-expanded lung tissue. It is usually recommended that not more than 1·0-1·5 l is aspirated at one time. If the lung is unable to re-expand freely a high negative intrapleural pressure may develop as fluid is aspirated. This will be felt by the operator as an increased pull on the syringe plunger and by the patient as chest tightness accompanied by coughing. Both of these complications can be relieved by letting air into the pleural space to lower the negative pressure, but this delays re-expansion of the lung and may permit loculation of the fluid.

In the absence of a clotting defect pleural aspiration rarely leads to serious haemoptysis or haemothorax. The former may occur if pleural biopsy is attempted without first obtaining fluid and the latter if the vessels at the lower border of the rib are damaged. Pneumothorax can result if the needle tip penetrates the visceral pleura or if air is inadvertently allowed to enter via the needle. If the pneumothorax is large an intercostal drain with underwater seal may be required. If the aspiration needle tears the visceral pleura and a superficial vein, air may be sucked into the pulmonary veins from the needle itself or from the adjacent lung. The air may enter any systemic artery, most often the cerebral vessels, and produce transient neurological symptoms and signs. The customary emergency treatment is to tilt the patient head down and with his right side uppermost to reduce the chance of air entering these arteries. Many deaths previously certified as "pleural shock" were probably due to air embolus, but vagal inhibition can also occur. Empyema after a non-sterile aspirating technique is rare, but nevertheless infection may be introduced and convert a sterile pleural effusion into a difficult empyema. Possible complications in cases of mesothelioma have already been mentioned.

LIVER BIOPSY

J R F WALTERS   A PATON

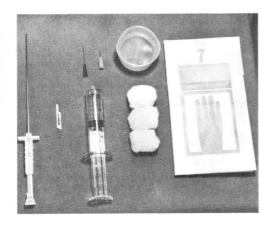

Percutaneous needle biopsy of the liver is a simple bedside procedure that provides a core of tissue for laboratory investigation and so is valuable in many types of liver disease and systemic illness. Several different instruments are available, each with its own technique. The general principles apply to all, but our discussion of procedure is confined to the disposable Tru-cut needle. Liver biopsy may also be carried out at laparotomy and laparoscopy and transvenously, but we do not propose to discuss these methods.

A blind procedure in an organ as vascular as the liver can be hazardous, so physicians should be well prepared and rehearsed. Practice with the appropriate instrument may be got in the necropsy room, but there is no substitute for learning by watching and copying someone who performs liver biopsies every week.

Indications

Cirrhosis

Hepatitis

Tumours

"Difficult" jaundice

Drug effects

Hepatomegaly

(1) Confirmation of a clinical diagnosis of cirrhosis.

(2) Investigation of chronic hepatitis and assessment of the effects of treatment.

(3) Histological confirmation of primary and secondary tumours.

(4) Investigation of "difficult" jaundice.

(5) Investigation of the effects of drugs, including alcohol, on the liver.

(6) Occasionally in acute hepatitis and hepatomegaly, and when liver function tests give abnormal results that remain unexplained.

(7) As an aid to diagnosing pyrexia of undetermined origin, granulomatous disease, and lymphomas.

Liver biopsy

Considerations

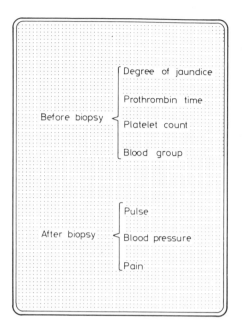

Before biopsy
- Degree of jaundice
- Prothrombin time
- Platelet count
- Blood group

After biopsy
- Pulse
- Blood pressure
- Pain

Can the patient understand the procedure and hold his breath for five seconds?—A violent cough or gasp when the needle is in position may tear the liver, with disastrous bleeding. A general anaesthetic is usually required in children.

Is the patient likely to bleed excessively?—The prothrombin time is the best indication: if it is prolonged more than three seconds and biopsy is considered to be essential then fresh-frozen plasma should be given (one unit before, one during, and one after the biopsy); if it is over six seconds the procedure should not be carried out. When the prothrombin time is abnormal 10 mg of vitamin K may be given parenterally for a few days. The platelet count is less important, but if it is below $50 \times 10^9/1$ (50 000/mm^3) care should be taken; platelet concentrates may be used. The patient's blood group should be known, and one unit of cross-matched blood should be available.

Is the path to the liver normal?—Biopsy is best postponed when there is a skin or chest infection. Ascites causes the liver to float away from an advancing needle and when appreciable should be treated first.

Is biopsy likely to do more harm than good?—Patients with deep jaundice, especially from extrahepatic obstruction, risk biliary peritonitis as well as haemorrhage, and if cholangitis is present the infection may be spread. Consider the possibility of a hydatid cyst, when anaphylaxis may result, or a vascular tumour including hepatoma, when angiography may be a better investigation.

Procedure

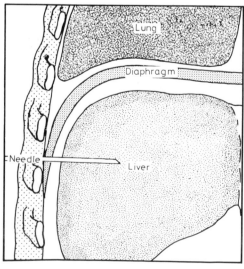

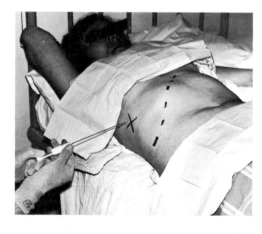

The patient lies along the edge of the bed with his right arm behind his head, which is turned to the left. A pillow placed firmly along the left side of the body will keep it horizontal. Palpate the abdomen and percuss the liver in the mid-axillary line: remember that it is largely intrathoracic. Mark the rib space which is below the top of the liver dullness on full expiration. It may be helpful to mark the xiphisternum and liver edge as well.

Sedation is not usually necessary, but plenty of local anaesthetic is. Draw up 10 ml of 1% lignocaine. Clean the skin with methylated spirit, and anaesthetise through a 25-gauge needle with a few drops of lignocaine in the appropriate space just above the rib. Then, using a 21-gauge needle, anaesthetise the deeper tissues with the patient breathing quietly, and advance slowly until a scratchy sensation or a gasp of pain indicates the sensitive tissues overlying the liver. Infiltrate this area with large amounts of anaesthetic. Remove the needle and, if you wish, measure the approximate distance to the surface of the liver on the biopsy needle.

Instruct the patient on how to take several deep breaths in and out and how to hold his breath in deep expiration for as long as he can. When you are satisfied that he understands, nick the skin with the point of a scalpel blade, introduce the biopsy needle, and advance slowly with the patient breathing quietly. If you are not sure of the depth of the liver surface, continue advancing until the needle begins to swing with respiration, then withdraw slightly until it stops swinging.

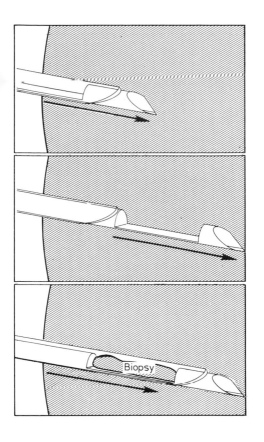

Repeat the breathing instructions with the patient following you. As soon as the breath is held in expiration thrust the *closed* needle about an inch into the liver. Advance the inner trocar, holding the outer cutting sheath still. Fix your right elbow against your side (to prevent the instinctive desire to withdraw the needle), advance the outer cutting sheath to cut the liver in the biopsy notch, and quickly withdraw the whole needle from the patient. With practice this sequence should take only a second or two. We prefer it to the one recommended by the manufacturer, as do others we have consulted, because it ensures that the specimen is taken from within the liver rather than from under the capsule.

Cover the skin incision with a plaster and instruct the patient to lie on the right side for four hours and to remain in bed for 24 hours. Pulse rate and blood pressure should be recorded hourly, and nurses instructed to report at once any alteration in condition or any complaint of pain.

Remove the biopsy specimen from the notch and divide it if specimens are needed for bacterial culture, biochemical examination, or electron microscopy in addition to histological examination. Place the histological specimen in formol saline on a piece of card to prevent fragmentation. Record the procedure in the notes, together with the texture and naked-eye appearance of the biopsy specimen: fat, pigmentation, tumour, and cirrhosis can sometimes be recognised.

What can go wrong

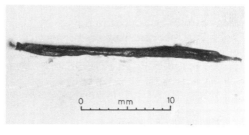

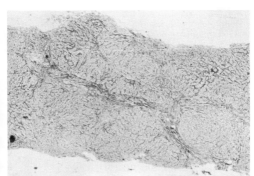

No liver tissue is obtained—This occurs most commonly when the sequence of movements is incorrectly performed, the inner trocar being withdrawn when the outer sheath should have been advanced. Incorrect positioning (as in very fat people, when it may be difficult to outline liver dullness), inadequate expiration, or a small or mobile liver are other reasons. The experienced performer permits himself no more than two attempts at biopsy.

Severe pain may be caused by bleeding or leakage of bile. Shoulder-tip pain and discomfort over the site of biopsy when the effect of the local anaesthetic wears off may require simple analgesia. Anything more than this should always be reported and patient and nurses instructed accordingly Biliary peritonitis is fortunately rare, but if in doubt seek a surgical opinion.

Shock is usually caused by rapid loss of blood from a large vessel or vascular tumour, less often by Gram-negative septicaemia. Bleeding may be more insidious, and blood transfusion should be started if there is unexplained tachycardia or hypotension, and fresh-frozen plasma or platelets given if indicated. Rarely, surgical intervention will be needed.

Septicaemia may result from needling an infected bile duct or liver abscess and may be the first indication of infection.

Rarer complications include haemoptysis or pneumothorax owing to biopsy of the lung, and biliary or bacterial peritonitis owing to puncture of gall bladder or colon respectively.

ARTERIAL PUNCTURE

D C FLENLEY

Indications

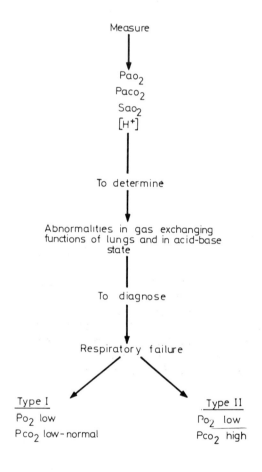

Arterial puncture is carried out in order to measure the arterial blood-gas tensions (Pao_2 and $Paco_2$), oxygen saturation (Sao_2), and pH (or [H^+]) so as to determine (1) abnormalities in the gas exchanging function of the lungs, for which it is necessary to know also the concentration of oxygen being inspired at the time of puncture; and (2) the patient's acid-base state, by relating the $Paco_2$ to the pH (or [H^+]), both to diagnose a disorder and as a guide to its treatment.

Arterial puncture is thus essential for the accurate diagnosis of respiratory failure, which may have been suspected clinically by noting central cyanosis. Only by knowing arterial blood-gas tensions can the type of respiratory failure be identified—for example, type I with a low Po_2 and normal or low Pco_2; or type II, in which a low Po_2 is associated with a high Pco_2. As the management of these two conditions may differ considerably, accurate diagnosis is essential.

Although measurement of the venous bicarbonate concentration will give some indication of the severity of a *metabolic* acid-base disturbance, definition of the type and severity of a *respiratory* acid-base disturbance can be made only when arterial Pco_2 and pH (or [H^+]) are known.

Contraindications

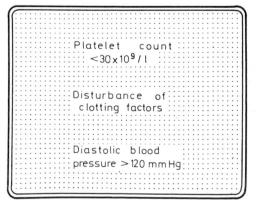

Contraindications to arterial puncture include a bleeding diathesis, as for example a platelet count below $30 \times 10^9/1$ (30 000/mm^3); and disturbance of clotting factors as in haemophilia and hypoprothrombinaemia or after overdoses of anticoagulants such as heparin, etc. In these conditions arterial puncture may lead to an excessive local haematoma, and this may also rarely complicate arterial puncture in patients with a diastolic blood pressure over 120 mm Hg.

Site of puncture

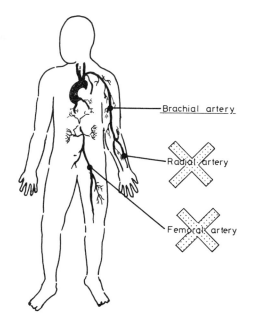

The brachial artery, just above the elbow crease, of the non-dominant arm—that is, the left arm in a right-handed person—is preferred. Patients are used to blood sampling at this site, where the artery is usually easily palpated, and personal experience shows that a small haematoma in the antecubital fossa is not painful, in contrast to a similar-sized haematoma after puncture of the radial artery at the wrist. Puncture of the femoral artery in the groin is not advised, as this site is embarrassing to the patient, inconvenient for the operator, and not infrequently yields blood from the femoral vein, which is much larger than the accompanying femoral artery—an error that can lead to potentially grave mistakes in diagnosis and treatment.

Equipment

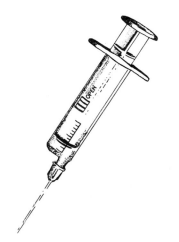

(1) Equipment for skin preparation (swabs, 1% cetrimide, etc).

(2) Some 1% plain lignocaine (without adrenaline) contained in a 5 ml syringe fitted with an orange (25 G) needle for local anaesthesia. This is *always* required—anyone who doubts this should be subjected to arterial puncture without it! The arterial puncture is carried out with a sterile all-glass, heavily-siliconised 10-ml syringe, in which the barrel moves easily. This syringe contains a stainless-steel washer, and the dead space is filled with a solution of heparin containing 1000 units/ml. The syringe is fitted with a green (21 G) disposable needle with a conventional bevel.

(3) Two or three 7·5 cm gauze swabs, and a 7·5 cm crêpe bandage.

Procedure

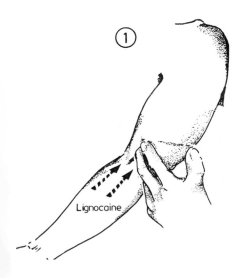

Outpatients should be seated, and the left arm may easily be supported on the edge of the consulting desk, to hyperextend the arm at the elbow. In patients in bed the arm may be hyperextended on a pillow. It is essential to make sure that the brachial artery can be palpated, the artery usually lying slightly medial to the tendon of the biceps at the top of the antecubital fossa. After skin preparation 0·5-1·0 ml of the local anaesthetic is infiltrated on each side of the artery and then, as the needle is withdrawn, a small bleb left just under the skin. To prevent injection of lignocaine into the artery it is advisable always to attempt to withdraw fluid into the syringe before injecting at any site. If this withdrawal yields bloodstaining the needle point should be moved before the local anaesthetic is injected.

The patient should be warned that he may have some tingling and numbness in the hand, which may last for 30-60 minutes after puncture, but that this results from partial anaesthesia of the median nerve, which lies very close to the brachial artery in the antecubital fossa. This symptom is of no clinical consequence.

Arterial puncture

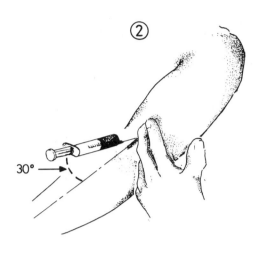

After leaving two to three minutes for the local anaesthetic to act use the arterial puncture syringe, with a green (21 G) 3·8 cm (1·5 in) needle attached, to obtain the sample of arterial blood. With the bevel upwards the needle is advanced through the skin bleb of local anaesthetic towards the pulsations of the brachial artery, which is continuously palpated by two fingers of the operator's left hand. The syringe is held with the needle at some 30° or so to the skin surface and is advanced proximally almost to touch the surface of the humerus. The syringe is then steadily withdrawn while slight suction is maintained on the plunger. At some point blood will suddenly enter the syringe, when suction and movement of the syringe should cease. With the syringe held still the blood must be seen to *pulsate into the syringe under its own power*. This is the only proof of successful arterial puncture. As arterial puncture is usually carried out in patients with central cyanosis, in whom even arterial blood will appear bluish, the colour of the blood is never a reliable indicator that arterial, and not venous, blood is being sampled. Without moving the syringe gentle suction is then continued until a 5-6 ml sample is obtained, but suction should then again cease to reaffirm that blood is still pulsating into the syringe.

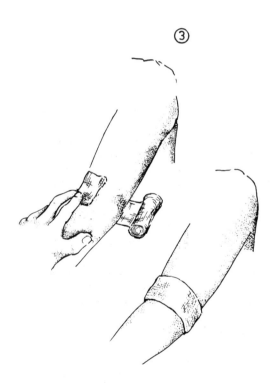

A folded 7·5 cm gauze swab is then firmly applied with the left hand over the puncture site and the needle and arterial puncture syringe completely withdrawn. The syringe is laid aside and firm pressure maintained over the puncture site through the gauze swab. This swab is then held firmly in position by a 7·5 cm crêpe bandage wrapped around the arm, each turn of the bandage being tightened. This firm bandage pressure, which will usually cause the arm below the bandage to become blue owing to obstruction of venous return, is maintained for five minutes. At the end of this time it is the responsibility of the operator to ensure that the bandage is removed.

After the bandage has been applied the syringe containing the arterial blood is taken in the right hand, with the plunger supported in the palm to prevent it from falling out. The needle is removed, and the one or two discrete air bubbles (all that are permitted) gently expelled by tapping the side of the syringe and pushing the plunger upwards so as to expel some blood into a swab held over the tip of the syringe. The syringe is then capped and gently inverted two or three times to allow the stainless-steel washer within the syringe to mix the sample.

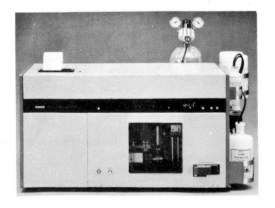

The sample is then taken directly to be injected into the blood-gas electrodes from the syringe without transfer to any other container. Blood-gas analysis should be carried out within five or not more than 10 minutes of removing the sample from the patient, and the sample should not be cooled during this period. If a greater delay is inevitable cooling the syringe and its contents in ice, with subsequent rewarming to body temperature before analysis, may help to minimise errors caused by continued metabolism of the white cells within the blood sample. This, however, is a compromise that is undesirable in practice, and measurement within five minutes of sampling is much preferred for accurate results.

The patient is warned that he may have a small haematoma over the site of puncture the following day. A useful way of expressing this is to say, "You may have a small bruise there tomorrow—if you do you will know that I am an honest doctor, and if you don't you may even think I'm a good one." Most patients appreciate such a comment.

Arterial puncture should be almost painless and thus not provoke hyperventilation due to anxiety or pain, which would tend to lower the Pco_2 and increase pH (lower hydrogen ion concentration), so adding a spurious temporary respiratory alkalosis to any other acid-base disturbance.

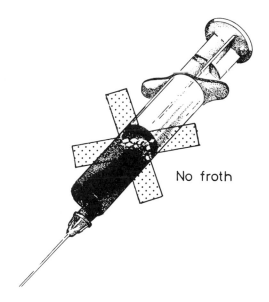

No froth

The syringe must be well lubricated by the heparin solution and have siliconised walls to ensure that the barrel moves easily under the patient's own pulsatile arterial blood pressure. The needle must fit tightly, and only very slight suction is applied, to prevent a froth of air and blood from forming within the syringe, which invalidates the anaerobic sample and makes the measurement meaningless. One or at most two small discrete bubbles are permitted, but these should be promptly expelled after the puncture as described above.

Recently Radiometer introduced a special arterial blood-gas sampling syringe (B109), which appears to be a useful method of obtaining a small sample of arterial blood suitable for use with the new automatic microsample blood-gas electrode systems. A similar special syringe is made by Concord Laboratories (Pulsator). Nevertheless, I prefer a larger sample, as this allows the measurements to be duplicated on the same sample, thus increasing confidence in the results.

Interpretation of results

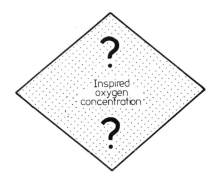

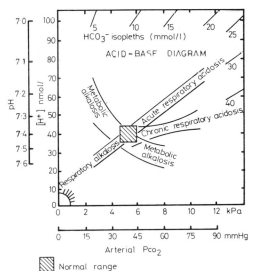

Normal range

Significance bands of single disturbances in human whole blood in vivo

To use arterial blood-gas analysis to measure any abnormality in the gas exchange function of the lungs it is essential that the approximate concentration of inspired oxygen at the time of withdrawing the arterial sample should be known. For example, with nasal prongs giving 2 l oxygen/min this concentration is about 30%; with the Ventimask (35%, 28%, 24%) the concentration is known more accurately, although most patients tolerate any masks less than the nasal prongs. With high-concentration oxygen treatment, as with the Polymask, 6 l oxygen/min delivers about 60% oxygen. At sea level the inspired oxygen tension (PIo_2) is then 60 kPa for 60% inspired oxygen, 30 kPa for 30% inspired oxygen, etc.

The alveolar to arterial oxygen-tension gradient ($A\text{-}aDo_2$) can then be estimated at the bedside, assuming that the patient's gas exchange ratio (R) is 1·0-0·8, which is usually true in most clinical circumstances.

Then, approximately,

$$PAo_2 = PIo_2 - \frac{Paco_2}{R}$$

$$A\text{-}aDo_2 = PAo_2 - Pao_2$$

where PAo_2 = calculated value of alveolar oxygen tension, PIo_2 = tension of inspired oxygen, $Paco_2$ = measured value of arterial Pco_2, and Pao_2 = measured value of arterial Po_2. In a normal adult at sea level, breathing air at rest, $A\text{-}aDo_2$ does not exceed 3·5 kPa (26 mm Hg). Normal arterial Pco_2 is 5·0-5·5 kPa (38-41 mm Hg), and arterial Po_2 10-14 kPa (75-105 mm Hg).

Acid-base disturbances can be characterised by the relations between the measured $Paco_2$ (or $[H^+]$) by plotting these values on an acid-base diagram, which is based on the empirically observed relations between these variables in the arterial blood of human patients with disease.

The photograph of the Radiometer ABL-2 blood-gas analyses is reproduced by permission of V A Howe and Co Ltd; the acid-base diagram is reproduced from the *British Journal of Hospital Medicine* by kind permission of the editor.

EAR SYRINGING

STUART CARNE

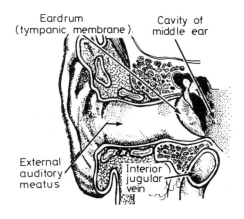

Wax (cerumen) is the secretion of the glands in the outer third of the external auditory meatus. Its consistency may be affected by atmospheric pollution. Normally it is expelled by ordinary chewing movements, but in some patients this does not happen. The wax then accumulates and may eventually block the external auditory meatus.

Indications

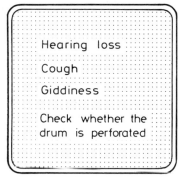

Symptomatic—(1) Hearing loss. (*a*) Acute onset: water in the ear may cause sudden swelling of the wax (for example, when swimming under water), which brings the patient rapidly to the doctor. (*b*) Gradual onset: the hearing loss may go unnoticed by the patient for a long time. (2) Earache: when the wax is pressing on the drum. (3) Cough: when the wax is pressing on the auricular branch of the vagus nerve. (4) Giddiness: sometimes present when there is an obstruction by wax in one meatus only.

Asymptomatic—Wax is frequently seen on routine examination. If the examination is for an insurance or pre-employment medical it may be necessary to remove the wax to ascertain whether (*a*) the hearing is normal and (*b*) the drum is perforated. Plugs of wax that do not block the meatus (and hence cannot affect the hearing) and still enable the drum to be seen may safely be left. Sometimes a thin film of wax on the drum (not painful) may give the impression that there is a perforation.

Note—The ordinary process of syringing when the middle ear is not inflamed often causes a temporary redness of the drum, which may confuse the diagnosis.

Contraindications

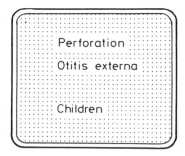

The presence of a perforation is a contraindication. Unfortunately, many patients are unaware of the perforation and it may not be identified until after the ear has been syringed. If necessary a prophylactic antibiotic should be administered systemically. Otitis externa is usually regarded as a contraindication because water can aggravate it. Nevertheless, many experienced doctors still syringe the ears when this condition is present but would always be careful gently to mop the meatus dry and might also instil some steroid drops (for example, betamethasone valerate lotion) twice daily for three or four days after syringing.

Wax in the ears of children poses special problems. Syringing the ears in a child is never easy and is particularly difficult when the child is ill. Nor is the procedure free from risk of trauma, especially if the child is fractious. Many experienced practitioners prefer to treat the suspected diagnosis rather than risk physical and emotional trauma.

Equipment

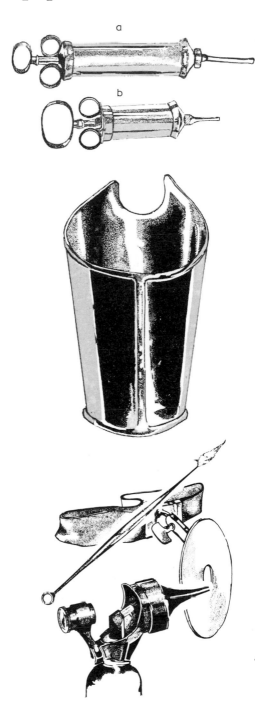

Syringe—Most ear syringes are about 18 cm long excluding the nozzle and hold about 120 ml of water (a). Shorter syringes are available (b): though they hold less water they are easier to balance. A plastic syringe of this latter design is produced by Russell Instruments, Glasgow. Some operators have found that a Water Pik (Teledyne Water Pik, Cranford, Middlesex), which is normally used in dentistry, is equally useful for syringing ears. Alternatively, a Higginson syringe may serve the purpose. Whatever instrument is used, sterility is not necessary.

Water—Plain tap water may be used and should be at or slightly above body temperature. The use of sodium bicarbonate in the water is not essential. Water that is too hot or too cold will stimulate the semicircular canals and may cause vertigo, nausea, and vomiting.

Towels—Traditionally a rubber or plastic apron is wrapped round the patient's neck to protect his clothes. The cost of laundering cloth towels normally prohibits their use, but paper towels are a satisfactory substitute. They may be tucked inside the collar and will soak up most, if not all, of any water that spills.

Collecting bucket—A Noot's tank is the most convenient, but if one is not available a kidney dish will do. The main disadvantage of the kidney dish is its habit of tipping over when partly full.

Wax hook—A wax hook (Jobson-Horne) is useful to lift out a plug of wax that remains obstinately in sight but keeps falling back or one that is stuck to the side wall of the meatus. In most patients experienced operators can remove all the ear wax with a hook without recoursing to syringing.

Lighting—A source of light, either a battery auriscope or a lamp, speculum, and head mirror, is essential for examining the ear before, during, and after the procedure. If a wax hook is to be used in the depths of the external auditory meatus a head mirror and speculum have an advantage over an electric auriscope in leaving one hand completely free to manipulate the hook.

Wax-softening agents—It is usually possible to syringe wax from an ear without any preparation, but first softening the wax eases the process. Sodium bicarbonate eardrops are effective. Alternatively, olive or almond oil or one of the proprietary preparations may be used. After any of these have been used for two to five days syringing may sometimes not be necessary. Some of the proprietary preparations, however, may cause otitis externa.

Procedure

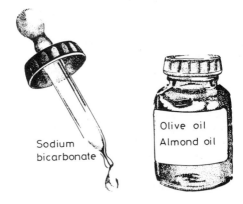

Sodium bicarbonate

Olive oil
Almond oil

If the indications for removing wax are not urgent, prescribe a suitable solvent to be used in the affected ear(s) night and morning for two to five days and ask the patient to return at the end of that time. Alternatively, an immediate attempt to remove the wax may be made with a hook or by syringing the ear without preparation. There is some evidence that using a solvent solution for even half an hour before syringing may offer some benefit.

Ear syringing

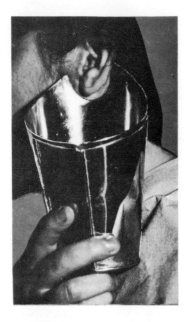

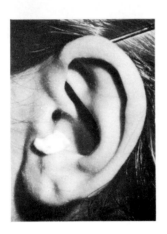

Have the patient sit comfortably in a chair, with his coat removed and a paper towel or plastic apron wrapped round his neck. The patient's co-operation is highly desirable if the meatus and drum are not to be damaged and water is not to be squirted all over the patient, the operator, and the rest of the room. Ask the patient to hold the Noot's tank below the ear, slotting the lobe into the groove. It is easier if the patient holds the tank to the right ear with the left hand and vice versa. This also reduces the risk of the patient knocking the operator's arm away.

When all is ready fill the syringe with water. Be sure no air remains in the syringe, as the sound of bubbles may be frightening to the patient. Pull the pinna up and back to straighten the external meatus. Put the tip of the nozzle at the edge of the external auditory meatus, pointed in the direction of the eardrum but slightly backward and downward (toward the patient's occiput). Some operators squirt the water in short bursts, others empty each syringeful in one or two actions. The jet of water should pass behind the wax and return into the tank. Sooner or later it will bring with it the lump of wax either intact or in fragments (often several large fragments: hence the need to inspect the ear during the procedure to ensure that all the wax has been cleared).

Water remaining in the meatus will restrict the view and should be gently mopped out with a pledget of cotton-wool or paper tissue, but do not damage the eardrum in trying to make sure that the ear is perfectly dry. A small pledget of cotton-wool may be left between the tragus and antitragus to mop up the last drops, but do not block the meatus.

When the first ear has been freed of wax turn the patient round slowly in his chair (rapid movement may make him giddy) and proceed in the same way with the other ear.

Complications

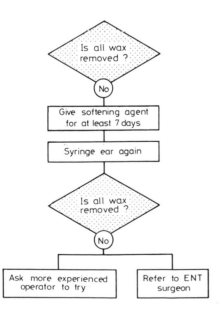

The most experienced operators sometimes fail to remove all the wax, even in the most co-operative patient and after using a softening agent. If the wax cannot be removed first time have the patient continue to use the softening agent for at least another seven days before repeating the procedure. If it again fails, ask a more experienced operator to try; alternatively, refer the patient to an ENT surgeon. Rarely, a general anaesthetic may be necessary.

If the meatus is scratched it will bleed. This is particularly likely to occur if a wax hook is used by an inexperienced operator. The blood should be gently mopped up with cotton-wool. Otitis externa is always a risk, but this may be reduced by careful drying (described above). If an already affected meatus is syringed the local application of steroid drops for one or two days after syringing reduces the risk of any further exacerbation.